Equine and Animal Reiki

Equine and Animal Reiki

Energy Healing for Horses and Family Pets

Randy Wilson

Copyright © 2023 Randy Wilson.

All rights reserved. No part of this publication may be reproduced, stored in a retrieval system or transmitted in any form or by any means—electronic, mechanical, photocopying, and recording or otherwise without the prior written permission of the author. To perform any of the above is an infringement of copyright law.

To the best of our knowledge, the content of this book provides accurate information that was correct at press time. The publisher and author assume no responsibility for errors, inaccuracies, omissions, or any other inconsistencies herein and hereby disclaim any liability to any party for any loss, damage, or disruption caused by errors or omissions, whether such errors or omissions result from negligence, accident, or any other cause.

The situations described are real and accurate. All photographs are for the sole purpose of illustrating the subject matter. Photographs taken at private stables or for private individuals have had their names, horse's names, and identifying details omitted or changed.

Photography Copyright © 2022 Randy Wilson; Kelly Poulin; Vicki Bennett.
Illustrations and diagrams Copyright © 2022 Randy Wilson.
Cover design Copyright © 2022 Jess Estrella.
Professional portrait taken by Cesar Correia; Copyright © 2022 Randy Wilson.

ISBN – 978-1-7775763-0-1 (Paperback)

1 2 3 4 5 6 7 8 9 10

First Printing, 2023

Published in Canada, by ReikiMaster Press

www.OttawaReikiMaster.com

Dedication

I dedicate this book to you, Carrington. You hold a very special place in my heart, like no other animal has before or probably ever will. You were my first horse client, my patient teacher, my mentor. You are such a gentle soul and I miss you dearly. You are still my inspiration for every Animal Reiki session I do. I feel your presence whenever I give a Reiki session to a horse.

Note to the Reader

The publisher and author make no guarantees concerning the level of success you may experience by following the advice and strategies contained in this book. Being near horses can be an inherently dangerous activity. The publisher and author assume no responsibility for your safety if you attempt any of these activities. This book is not intended as a substitute for professional medical or veterinary advice or treatment. The reader should consult a medical professional where appropriate.

Table of Contents

Acknowledgements..xii

Introduction..xiv

PART 1: An Introduction to Reiki...xix

Chapter 1: The Basics of Reiki..21
    What is Reiki?..21
    The Five Spiritual Principles of Reiki...................................22
    Learning to Do Reiki..23
    The Reiki Symbols..25
    Usui Reiki Is Just Reiki..25

Chapter 2: Your Path to Reiki Begins with You.......................27

Chapter 3: Energy and Chakras..31
    What Is Energy?..31
    What Are Chakras?...34
    Chakras 1, 2, and 3..35
    Chakra 4..36
    Chakras 5, 6 and 7...36
    Bud Chakras..38
    Brachial Chakra...38
    Other Important Chakras...39
    A Note About the Third Eye Chakra...................................39

PART 2: Guidelines for Treating Animals................................43

Chapter 4: Energy and Animals..45
    Ethics..47
    Do I Get a Treat for Accepting This?..................................48
    The Right Way to Approach It...48

PART 3: Doing the Healing Session..................................51

Chapter 5: Preparing Yourself for the Session..................53

    Preparing Your Mindset..53

    The Ego..54

    Rein In Your Energy..55

    Meditation..56

    Grounding..59

Chapter 6: Doing the Session...61

    A Few Reminders...61

    What Will This Be Like for Me?.......................................63

    The Sensations You May Feel..64

    The Best Time and Place for a Session...........................65

    On the Way to the Stable..66

    Your Personal Check-In..67

    Clearing the Space for the Session..................................69

    Asking Your Guides for Their Help...................................71

    Asking Permission, Offering Reiki....................................73

    Beginning the Session..76

    Following the Horse's Lead..77

    Hand Positions...78

    What Reactions You Might See.......................................88

    Wait, That's Just Way Too Intense!..................................92

    But I Don't Want You There..94

    Heart to Heart..95

    A Crying Horse...95

    Treating Horses in a Stall...96

    Treating Horses Tied to a Hitching Post..........................97

    Treating Horses in a Sand Ring, Arena, or Dry Pen.................98

    Treating Horses in a Pasture..99

    Treating Horses Outside, with Others Nearby........................100

    Time for Another Horse..101

    When to End a Session...102

    How to End a session...103

    Remind Me of What Just Happened....................................105

    Distance Sessions..105

Chapter 7: Ways to Enhance a Session.................................109

    Chakra Balancing..109

    Crystals...111

    Animal Communication..114

Chapter 8: Safety for You and the Horse..............................117

    My Space, Your Space, Our Space......................................119

    Going Toe-to-Toe with One Thousand Pounds....................121

    Sunny Days...122

    Can I Close My Eyes?..123

    In a Horse's Stall...126

    Outside a Horse's Stall..127

    At Liberty..127

    While Asleep..128

    Bio-security..131

    In the Age of COVID-19 and Beyond..................................134

PART 4: An Understanding of Horses....................................137

Chapter 9: Introducing my Mentor..139

Chapter 10: Understanding Horses.......................................143

    Horses' Zone of Awareness..145

Horses' Mental and Emotional States..........146

Chapter 11: Herd Dynamics and Reiki..........151

Can I Hang Out with Your Herd?..........151

To Share or Not to Share, That Is the Question..........154

Getting My Hands on Fire..........162

PART 5: Bonus Material for Equine Reiki..........167

Chapter 12: Frequently Asked Questions..........169

What Is a Typical Session Like?..........169

Is This a Good Time for a Session?..........170

Why Won't My Horse Accept My Reiki?..........170

I Am Really Short—How Can I Do This?..........171

Are You in Pain?..........172

But I Need You Now, Can I Go First?..........173

What Should I Wear When Conducting a Session?..........173

Can I Wear Jewelry?..........174

Can I Carry an Umbrella if It's Raining?..........174

Can There Be Music Playing During a Session?..........175

Can Two People Work on the Same Horse at Once?..........176

Can You Draw Reiki Symbols on Horses and Other animals?..........177

What if Another Horse Unintentionally Absorbs Some Reiki?..........177

How Do You Deal with Bugs and Insects at a Stable?..........178

How Can Reiki Help Therapy horses?..........179

Can Horses Be Reiki Practitioners?..........180

What Do I Do When Nothing Works?..........182

Why Do I Get Tired?..........183

Do I Need Business Insurance to Offer Reiki to Horses?..........184

Where Can I Find a Practitioner?..........185

- Where Can I Find Potential Clients?..186

Chapter 13: A Quick Checklist..189
- The Checklist:..189

PART 6: Treating Other Animals..193

Chapter 14: House Pets..195
- Your House Pets..195
- Reiki and House Pets..196
- A Pet's Emotional/Psychological State..199
- Ending a Session..201
- A Symbiotic Relationship..201

Chapter 15: Transitioning/End of Life..205

Chapter 16: Reiki and Other Animals..209
- Down on the farm..209
- At the Animal Shelter..210
- Wild Animals and Other Forest Creatures..211
- Lions and Tigers and Wolves, Oh My!..212

Afterword..214
- A Few Parting Words..214

List of Figures..216

About the Author..220

Acknowledgements

This book was made possible with the help of many people, horses, and other animal clients. I could not have learned how to do this healing work for animals without the patient mentoring of all the animals I have had the privilege of working with. I have had many wonderful animals share their lives with me. It has been my honour, pleasure, and privilege to learn from them.

Many thanks to all the people who taught me lessons about horses along this journey.

A big thank you to my wife Kelly Poulin. She listened to all my ramblings these past few years while I was writing this book, learning how to publish it, and debating all the decisions I had to make along the way.

Cesar Correia took my professional portrait and I love it.

Jess Estrella designed a wonderful cover and colophon for the book.

A heartfelt thanks to everyone who contributed to the photography, including all the stable owners and horse guardians who allowed photos to be taken on their property and/or of their horses, as well as everyone who took photos for me.

Vicki Bennett graciously offered her horses, Bella and Zip Pow, to be my photographic models in some of the photos that she took of us for use in this book. Bella and Zip Pow were more than happy to pose for the camera.

Sue Solf at Foymount Farm Equine Retreat was instrumental in helping me get started on this path. I spent many a day hanging out with her wonderful herd and offering them Reiki sessions. Her horses were some of my early teachers. This is where I completed the numerous case studies that were required to be certified with the Canadian Reiki Association.

A very special thanks to my editor Erin Della Mattia. Her positive encouragement and assurances helped me tremendously. Her view of the big picture and the structure of the book was evident early on. The recommendations she made were always highly insightful and her reasons for them were very well explained. We had some wonderful interactions over how to explain or describe things. This book would not be as polished and refined without her talent. I actually had the sense right from our first contact that she was the right editor for this project.

Some photos were taken by the author on the premises of the Therapeutic Riding Association Ottawa-Carleton (otherwise known as "TROtt"). These photos are used with the permission of TROtt, who is the owner of the photographed horses and the operator of the facility. These photos are used only for illustration purposes. Their use does not represent an endorsement by TROtt or any of its directors, officers, employees, or volunteers of the content of this book and/or my Reiki practice and/or its associated methods and results.

Introduction

Equine and Animal Reiki: Energy Healing for Horses and Family Pets is a definitive resource on how to do Reiki sessions for horses. It is also an entertaining account of my journey through years of learning how to do this for horses. I am a Reiki Master Teacher who has spent most of my Reiki practice healing horses and house pets. Treating animals has become my passion; they give us so much and ask us for so little. They deserve everything we can do for them to improve their lives.

Reiki energy healing is a holistic, non-invasive method of treating many physical ailments and injuries. It can improve overall health, both physical and emotional. Animals suffer traumas just like people do, and these experiences can manifest in behavioural issues, anxiety, and stress. Horses are valuable companions and are invaluable for the work they do for us. Unfortunately, many horses get abused, traumatized, or just neglected. They get used by us, and when they can no longer perform the function that we want them to, they get discarded.

Reiki is gaining popularity as a complementary therapy for helping animals. It can help animals work through their trauma and overcome their anxiety. It is not a replacement for formal medical care or treatment, but can supplement it by creating an energy balance throughout the animal's body.

On a physical level it can help:
- Ease tight muscles or restricted movement
- Relieve pain
- Lower blood pressure
- Increase lymphatic flow
- Rid the body of toxins
- Speed up recovery after illnesses or competitions
- Speed up the healing of physical injuries
- Boost performance

On an emotional level it can help:
- Relax an animal
- Ease an animal's stress and anxiety
- Reduce stress and anxiety from travel or trailering
- Alleviate emotional or trust issues caused by prior trauma, abuse, or neglect
- Resolve behavioural issues that may be rooted in past trauma, abuse, or neglect
- Adjust animals to new environments, like a new home[1]
- Soothe anxiety around temporary displacement, like at a competition
- Lighten the pain of loss (of a guardian or favourite companion)

Horses can become stressed, ill, or injured, and can benefit from Reiki as much as people do. The first thing horses want to do in the morning is get out and run, but injuries can compromise their

---

[1] It takes about three months for a horse or family pet to settle into a new home, start to feel safe, and trust that it really is their new permanent home.

mobility. We may need to restrict them to their stall, where they will be cooped up day after day, which can add more stress, and they don't even get a choice. Wouldn't you like to help them cope with this? Isn't this the ideal time for a non-invasive, non-chemical, alternative therapy that can assist with their stress management and their physical recovery? Can you think of a better time for a Reiki session?

In the pages of this book, you will get highly useful knowledge and tools for effectively using Reiki to treat horses, including step-by-step instructions for how to conduct Reiki sessions. The lessons you will learn can also be applied to other animals, including your family pet. If you are a Reiki practitioner and you are considering offering your talents to horses or your pet, then this book is for you. Do you own horses, or just love them? Are you interested in equine health care? If you are curious about holistic healing options or alternative medicine for horses or other animals, then this book is for you.

My expertise in treating horses is rooted in my Reiki knowledge, experience, and ability, as well as countless hours of hands-on experience treating horses over many years. This book started as notes to myself after each session that I offered. My notes were to remind myself what I was learning, what worked, and just as importantly what didn't work as I interacted with different horses, at different times, and in different places. I quickly realized that I had amassed a wealth of insight that would be useful for others who might also want to do this wonderful work. So, my personal notes got polished and formalized, and this book was born.

I came to treating horses through the back door, as I say. I grew up in southern Ontario, with a menagerie of animals that included dogs, cats, hamsters, guinea pigs, mice, rabbits, ducks, budgies, pigeons, turtles, and even snakes. As you can guess, I developed a love for animals at an early age. When I initially learned Reiki, there was no doubt in my mind that I would continue on to the Reiki Master Teacher Level. Yet, despite growing up surrounded by animals, I never envisioned myself treating them.

My first equine client was Carrington. He was an injured elite jumper who could no longer carry a rider. I had recently finished my Reiki Master Teacher training and offered his guardian a session for him. She was open to this even though I had never worked on a horse before. Carrington was my initial teacher. Despite not being able to carry his weight evenly on all four legs he was very patient with me.

My Reiki Master Level gave me the ability and confidence that I could do this. To develop my knowledge further, I went looking for books on the subject. There are a bunch on Animal Reiki, but precious few specifically deal with Reiki for horses. I have read most of the ones I found. There are also many online videos that show people offering Reiki to animals, but few explain the entire process of doing it from start to finish. So, I invested time and energy in courses and workshops, including Animal and Equine Reiki; personal development topics related to enhancing intuition and psychic abilities; and Animal Communication. Much research, study, and practice taught me what reactions and behaviours to expect from my new animal clients and how to work with them safely. I think very few people have ever taught this, at least in my part of Canada, and nobody anywhere near my city. So, on top of offering Reiki to horses, I now teach Equine Reiki classes.

In addition to this work, I am certified as an Equine Assisted Learning (EAL) Personal Development Coach. There is a therapeutic riding association in my area with whom I regularly volunteer my time to provide their therapy horses with Reiki sessions. I am also an Animal Communicator, and there are references throughout this book about me talking to the animals I treat. You don't need this ability to be effective at treating animals with Reiki, but I will touch on it briefly since it goes hand-in-hand with many forms of energy healing like Reiki.

Once you start applying these healing techniques, the animals in your life will be happier and healthier than they ever were before. If you want to help your animal friends be the healthiest they can be, it's time to get started on your healing journey together, using Reiki.

PART 1: An Introduction to Reiki

Randy Wilson

Chapter 1: The Basics of Reiki

What is Reiki?

Usui Reiki is a Japanese system of energy healing that originated with the teachings of Mikao Usui. It is a non-invasive alternative healing method for reducing stress and improving overall health. I describe Reiki as a relaxing energy massage. It's a massage for your entire being, it's just done with energy, not with physical manipulation.

We well know any form of relaxation or stress relief helps improve health and well-being. Practitioners of Reiki understand that if the natural flow of energy through the body is weakened or blocked, it can manifest itself in stress and other physical symptoms. Reiki can increase and balance these energies and assist with many illnesses. It helps balance a body's energy field and energy centres, or chakras, to help maintain health. The original intent of Reiki was for self-development and self-improvement. It was only later that people realized they could use it as a healing modality for others. Reiki is quickly becoming accepted as an alternative holistic healing option and has been used in hospitals in the United States since the mid-1990s.[2]

Everyone can benefit from Reiki, including people, animals, plants, and even food (but don't expect it to turn unhealthy food into healthy food). It is useful for dealing with daily stresses such as anxiety, anger, or frustration, along with other chronic ailments. Reiki is not a replacement for medical treatment, but it does enhance the body's natural ability to heal itself.

Reiki can do no harm. It will not make an injury worse, although you may experience some discomfort during any healing process.

The Five Spiritual Principles of Reiki

- Just for today, I will not be angry.
- Just for today, I will not worry.
- Just for today, I will give thanks for my many blessings.
- Just for today, I will do my work honestly.
- Just for today, I will be kind to every living thing.

These are principles for guiding your life. None of us are expected to be perfect, and there is no final state for you to be in. That's why they all start with "Just for today."

---

[2] William Lee Rand, "Reiki in Hospitals," The International Center for Reiki Training, https://www.reiki.org/articles/reiki-hospitals.

Learning to Do Reiki

Reiki is quick, easy, and inexpensive to learn, and anyone can learn it. You just need to be attuned to the energy frequency and be taught how to connect to it and use it. The ability to channel Reiki energy is passed from a Reiki Master to a student through a process called an attunement. It consists of a deep healing session and will clear any energy blockages. It then connects the student to the Reiki energy frequency so they can then channel the energy through themselves to their clients.

Once you are attuned to Reiki it is always on, to some degree. We think of turning it on and off, but in fact your base energy frequency is slightly higher than it used to be. That means you always have some of it running. It is sitting in the background waiting for you to ask it to do something. When we "turn it on" we are just intentionally setting its intensity to its maximum. We are also placing ourselves in the right mental and emotional state to perform a Reiki treatment and to place our total focus on our client. Where our focus goes, energy goes.

Acquiring Reiki Level 1 (or first degree) gives you the ability to treat people or animals. Reiki Level 2 (or second degree) gives you the ability to do Reiki sessions from a distance. This is a wonderful ability to have when working on horses, especially in situations where physical contact or even being close could be a safety issue. For this reason, Reiki level 2 is the prerequisite for my Equine Reiki classes.

Many holistic clinics, physiotherapy clinics, health spas, and New Age shops could point you to a Reiki Teacher in your area. If you are in Canada, you can search the Canadian Reiki Association website for links to teachers in a city near you. Not all teachers in Canada are members, and some are only registered with the Association as practitioners. I was taught in my Master Teacher class that we should teach Reiki 1 and 2 in person, and that students should be attuned in person. Although there are many online Reiki classes on offer, for me there really is no substitute for learning from an experienced Master Teacher in person. They will do the attunement and teach you how to use the Reiki, as well as offer guidance and answer questions. Plus, you get to practise with your fellow students, who can give you instant feedback. You will see their reactions when you practise on them, and they will describe what they noticed when they practised on you. This gives you a wonderful connection to others in your area to practise with as you continue along your Reiki journey. It's also worth noting that to be registered as a Reiki practitioner or teacher with the Canadian Reiki Association you have to have taken your training in-person.

If you do choose to take an online class, I strongly recommend that it provide more than just the attunements. This is not enough. The course should include explanations, diagrams of hand placements, descriptions of how to perform a Reiki session, when to use Reiki, and when not to use it. It should teach you what sensations and reactions to expect from yourself and your client. It should include the ethics of doing this for others and provide access to the teacher to answer your questions.

Some teachers now teach levels 1 and 2 together, which I do not agree with. Each level is a starting point, not an endpoint. You are starting on a journey of understanding Reiki and learning how to use it effectively. It's not a race to the piece of paper that lets you take the next level. Energy is instantaneous, but your physical body is denser and takes about three weeks to adjust to the energy frequency shift that Level 1 will give you. Level 2 is a tremendous leap if you only got your Level 1 about ten minutes ago. You may not recognize the sensations yet or believe it is actually working. Use your Level 1 to give yourself the recommended twenty-one days of self-treatment. You need to believe that it is working and practice using it before considering taking your Level 2. My teacher taught me to wait three to six months between taking Level 1 and Level 2. Then to wait much longer before considering taking the Master Level.

The Reiki Symbols

There are three basic Reiki symbols. They are most often taught in Reiki Level 2, which is when I teach them. There is a power symbol named Cho Ku Rei (CKR), a mental/emotional symbol named Sei He Ki (SHK), and a distance symbol named Hon Sha Ze Sho Nen (HSZSN). The symbols are an image made of a sequence of lines drawn in a specific order. You can draw them on an object, in the air, or just visualize the symbol in your mind. Many people use the power symbol as their initial intent to connect to their Reiki energy (which many people think of as turning it on). The SHK symbol assists with or enhances mental and emotional issues. You use it (draw it) if the session is meant to enhance someone's ability to learn something or to help with emotional issues. The distance symbol is drawn during a session to help you make the connection to someone's energy when you are doing a distance session. They can all be used at once. The power symbol used with another symbol enhances its strength/intensity. You get attuned to them in your Reiki class; only then will they work for you.

Usui Reiki Is Just Reiki

This book is about using Usui Reiki to treat horses. There are many ways of doing anything, including energy healing. I do not suggest any of the other methods are less effective than Usui Reiki.

The Western world has recently created a multitude of variations of Reiki. That's fine; the world can use all the help it can get from anything that works.

If you are using Usui Reiki, you need no physical tools, equipment, plants, crystals, stars, celestial bodies, or anything else. You only need the Reiki to do what I am presenting here. Usui Reiki is just Reiki, and nothing else.

I use other forms of energy healing too. I will use crystals and other healing techniques and often combine them with Reiki in a session. You can enhance a Reiki session with whatever else works for you and combine it with anything else. Just remember that things like crystal healing are not specifically Reiki.

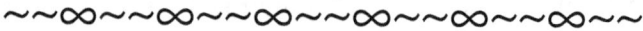

Summary

Anyone can learn Reiki. It is easy and inexpensive to learn. You can use it to treat yourself, other people, animals, and even your house plants. It doesn't require any tools, equipment, or celestial bodies—just you and your connection to the universal Reiki energy.

Chapter 2: Your Path to Reiki Begins with You

Learning Reiki is one path to a more enlightened and aware life. Doing energy healing requires you to confront you own issues, especially if you want to heal others. When you are channelling Reiki energy, you are a conduit for the energy. The energy flows through your body to the client. Since it passes through your body, you become a filter for the energy. It absorbs some of who you are on its way through. You don't want it picking up any negative, disturbing or disruptive energy patterns from you. You can't get clean, clear water by passing it through a dirty filter. You need to be the clearest channel possible. That's why you need to work on yourself first.

If you were to offer Reiki to others and, during a session, touch on the client's feelings of anger, sadness, or grief and then react to your own experience of it, this would not be conducive to helping your client. You can't be effective if you have strong or overwhelming personal reactions to someone else's issues. Therefore, doing emotional healing on yourself first can make you a more effective energy healer.

A very good understanding of what issues are yours will help you distinguish them from whatever you get from your client. Practising Reiki on yourself regularly will help you understand what is yours and what isn't.

You need to learn to leave your own issues at the door when you are treating people, but it is crucial when treating animals. Our pets pick up the negative energy that we project onto them. They come into our lives as companions, teachers, spiritual helpers, and healers. They will often and readily pick up our emotional state. Sometimes they even adopt our physical issues. If you approach an animal while in need of emotional healing yourself, she will sense it and want to help. Animals can't accept healing from you if they are trying to give it to you.

That's why I advise you to address your own issues and work on yourself first. You don't have to have it "all together" before you can do this. We are all works in progress.

To create an effective healing environment for your client, you need to hold a very high energy vibration that is stable, consistent, loving, and non-judgmental. The consensus is that Reiki Level 1 is best suited for treating yourself, your family members, and friends. Reiki Level 2 is considered the minimum level if you want to use it to help others or charge for your services. Presumably (and hopefully) by the time you get to your Reiki 2 you have already done many months of the recommended daily self-healing sessions. When I hear people say that the only reason they plan to learn Reiki is to "fix" this person or "fix" that pet, I think it is admirable, but I believe they are putting the cart before the horse. You always have to come first.

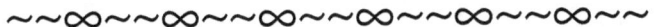

Summary

Reiki will improve your life in so many ways, even if you never use it to treat other people or animals.

Chapter 3: Energy and Chakras

What Is Energy?

How do you explain energy? If you mention the word energy to many people, they probably start thinking about their ability —or more often, inability—to do personal activities. *"I'm just too tired to go to the gym, do yoga, take that walk. I got very little sleep last night. I am so tired, a nap would be great. I wish I had as much energy as my toddler."* Sound familiar?

If you are not thinking like this, you may be remembering your high school science class. That's where you learned about the scientific approach to energy based on physical laws and mathematical equations for measuring it and its role in shaping our universe. You likely learned how to use formulas and scientific tools to measure different types of energy and then how to use that energy to create changes in the world through methods like steam power, electrical connections, and propulsion.

I am going to give you a different perspective on what energy is. Everything that exists is just energy. All forms of energy are connected to everything else, everywhere, all the time. We are in constant contact with many invisible forms of energy that enter our bodies, circulate through them, and then exit. The entire universe is just a collection of limitless frequencies of energy, all intertwined.

"Frequency" is a scientific term that describes how many events occur within a specific time frame. All forms of energy are vibrating in their own unique frequency range. The Earth itself vibrates with a specific energy frequency: it's called the Schumann Resonance (7.83 Hz). Most energy frequencies are not visible to us, like ultraviolet light, infrared light, or cellphone transmissions. Energy travels right through things that appear to be solid, like radio waves passing through the walls of your house.

Anything that is moving is energy, and everything is always moving. Everything in your physical reality is in constant motion: rocks, trees, dirt, plants, animals—everything. Even the chair you are sitting on is moving.

In this understanding of energy, you are not the physically separate body you think you are. Your body is a collection of energy, not solid or motionless but always in motion. Our bodies generate a constantly changing energy field that surrounds us like an invisible bubble, sometimes called your aura.

Energy flows through our bodies from head to toe and back again. This energy must move consistently, freely, and unobstructed through our bodies to keep them healthy. We can't work at peak efficiency if our energy is blocked or depleted anywhere along its natural path. If it is, then we will probably develop issues related to physical, emotional, psychological, or spiritual health.

Just as energy flows through our bodies, it also flows from one person to another. Once you get physically close to another person's energy field or aura, your energy merges and intermingles with theirs, and you become much more aware of your energetic connection to them. Every time you meet someone, there is an exchange of energy. It's like two batteries connecting: the weaker one naturally draws energy from the stronger one. This isn't to say that one person is "weaker" than the other. It's just that at that specific moment in time one person will be happier than the other, or more emotionally balanced, more grounded, more confident, physically healthier, or vibrating at a slightly higher frequency.

It is natural that the other person will absorb some of that energy for themselves. It's not deliberate, malicious, or even conscious. This is partly how energy healing works: you provide someone with loving, positive energy to absorb and use as they need. When you are doing a Reiki session, you are intentionally holding a higher frequency of energy than they are, so it naturally flows to them. Reiki is not something you do "to" someone. You do not "push" Reiki into them, they draw it from you.

In order to effectively offer energy healing to others, you also need to know how to avoid projecting your own personal energy or emotions onto others, including animals. You must stay conscious of the energy that is yours and the energy you may have picked up from others. Our bodies can hold on to energy that isn't ours. You need to know how to dissipate it so you don't hold on to it.

There is no such thing as empty space. You are not a physical body living "in" the universe, separate from all the other energy that exists. You are an integral part of all the energy that makes up the entire universe. To use another common analogy, you are a drop of water in the ocean. When you are in the ocean, you are indistinguishable from the totality of the ocean, so from a wider perspective you actually *are* the ocean. We are no longer separate physical beings; we are all just part of universal consciousness.

For doing energy healing work, all you really need to understand is that everything is connected on an energy level. This is what enables us to offer Reiki from a distance.

It is quite a revelation to think in terms of everyone and everything on the planet being connected. Once you get this awareness, you won't look at the world the same way again. Your entire view of reality shifts.

What Are Chakras?

The Sanskrit word "chakra" literally translates to wheel or disk. Chakras are energy centres that absorb universal energy and channel it through our bodies. The energy that makes up and maintains our existence has a physical, mental, emotional, and spiritual component. These must all stay in balance for us to be totally healthy.

Think of chakras as spinning wheels of energy. Each chakra vibrates at a slightly different frequency and has a specific purpose. Every chakra spins clockwise and resonates to its own colour and musical note. Each one corresponds to different mental, emotional, psychological, and spiritual functions, and to physical organs in the body.

Every chakra needs to stay open, with energy flowing through it unrestricted, to keep all aspects of your life in balance.

Depending on who you ask, there are hundreds of chakras. Much of the Western world knows of seven main chakras. Here is one common understanding of the seven-chakra system: root, sacral, solar plexus, heart, throat, third eye, and crown.

Chakras 1, 2, and 3

The first three chakras relate to your physical existence.

The first is the "root" chakra.
- Its colour is red.
- This chakra is at the base of your spine.
- It relates to your basic physical needs, existence, security, survival, and trust; it connects you to the earth.
- Physically it relates to the reproductive system and controls sexual development.
- The organs it corresponds to are the kidney and spine.
- Its corresponding phrases are: *"I have," "I am,"* and *"I am safe."*
- Changing a horse's environment or home can cause an imbalance to this chakra.

The second is the "sacral" chakra.
- Its colour is orange.
- This chakra is above your pubic bone and below your navel.
- It relates to your creativity, sexuality, self, well-being, and pleasure.
- Physically it relates to the immune system and metabolism.
- The organs it corresponds to are the adrenal gland, kidneys, gallbladder, bowel, and spleen.
- Its corresponding phrases are: *"I feel"* and *"I am creative."*
- Being isolated from his herd can affect a horse's sacral chakra.

The third is the "solar plexus" chakra.
- Its colour is yellow.
- This chakra is in the middle of your breastbone.
- It relates to your sense of personal power, self-confidence, self-esteem, control, and vital energy.

- Physically it relates to the regulation of metabolism.
- The organs it corresponds to are the intestines, pancreas, liver, bladder, and stomach.
- Its corresponding phrases are: "*I can,*" "*I do,*" and "*I am strong.*"
- Anything that makes a horse feel out of control can affect this one.

Chakra 4

The fourth is your "heart centre" chakra.
- Its colour is green.
- It is the connection between your bottom three physical chakras and your top three spiritual ones.
- It relates to your connection to love, joy, care, and emotions.
- Physically it regulates the immune system and circulatory system.
- The organs it corresponds to are the thymus, heart, and lungs.
- Its corresponding phrases are: "*I love*" and "*I am loved.*"
- Any physical or emotional abuse, any loss, or anything that makes a horse feel unwanted or unloved can affect this one.

Chakras 5, 6 and 7

The top three chakras relate to your spiritual existence.

The fifth is the "throat" chakra.
- Its colour is light blue.
- This chakra is at your throat, as the name suggests.
- It relates to your verbal expression and all communication.

- Physically it regulates body temperature, immunity, the respiratory system, and metabolism.
- The organ it corresponds to is the thyroid.
- Its corresponding phrases are: "*I speak*" and "*I am expressive.*"
- A horse's environment can affect this one, especially if it is not very natural (like total stall living, little or no turnout).

The sixth is the "third eye" chakra.
- Its colour is deep blue.
- This chakra is right between your eyebrows.
- It relates to your intuition, imagination, clairvoyance, psychic senses, and wisdom.
- Physically it regulates the nervous system and biological cycles, including sleep.
- The organ it corresponds to is the pineal gland.
- Its corresponding phrases are: "*I see*" and "*I am connected.*"
- Toxic or erratic energy can affect this one; horses are so aware of and in tune with the emotional state of their environment.

The seventh is the "crown" chakra.
- Its colour is deep purple or indigo.
- This chakra is on the crown of your head.
- It is the meeting point between your physical body and the universe (cosmic consciousness, your soul).
- It relates to your sense of enlightenment, your spiritual connection to the universe and divine source energy, awareness, intelligence, and cosmic consciousness.
- Physically it governs the functions of other glands and is responsible for growth.
- The organs it corresponds to are the central nervous system, pituitary gland, and spinal cord.

- Physical pain can affect this one, and emotional pain can too, since this chakra relates to the nervous system and one's sense of connection.
- Its corresponding phrases are: "*I know*," "*I understand*," and "*I am Divine.*"
- Having this chakra out of balance can cause a horse to be anxious and/or have trouble fitting into the herd.

Bud Chakras

All animals, including horses, have "bud" chakras, one on the bottom of each hoof or paw. These chakras keep horses grounded and create a connection to the earth. These very much relate to what the root chakra does.

Brachial Chakra

The "brachial" chakra is at the inside of the horse's shoulder, right beside the heart. This is a connection point between the horse and her guardian or foal. This is often where I start a session. Riding a horse without getting her permission first can affect this chakra. Poorly fitting saddles can cause back pain or pinched nerves. Having this chakra out of balance can cause the horse to resist letting you saddle or ride her.

Other Important Chakras

The earth star chakra is in the Earth, about eighteen inches below your feet. It grounds you to the Earth and to your physical existence. It connects directly to the core of the Earth (to Gaia).

The soul star chakra is about two feet above the crown chakra. It connects you to your soul's purpose.

A Note About the Third Eye Chakra

People who embark on a path of awakening often start by learning about chakras. I often hear people say things like "*I want to develop my psychic abilities,*" or "*I want to be more intuitive, or more spiritual, or connect with my guides.*" Since the third eye chakra plays an important role in psychic abilities, these people ask "*What do I have to do to open my third eye chakra?*" This focus on the third eye chakra is misplaced. You cannot function in this physical existence while being totally focused on your spiritual self. It doesn't work. You are living in a three-dimensional body. To have your third eye totally open, you must also have your root chakra effectively connecting you to your physical existence. They go hand in hand. Not only that, to be totally healthy you need all your chakras channelling energy through your body efficiently. They all have to be open equally. When you have them all open, you will have access to all that your third eye can provide you.

The diagram that follows indicates the placement of each of the chakras on a horse.

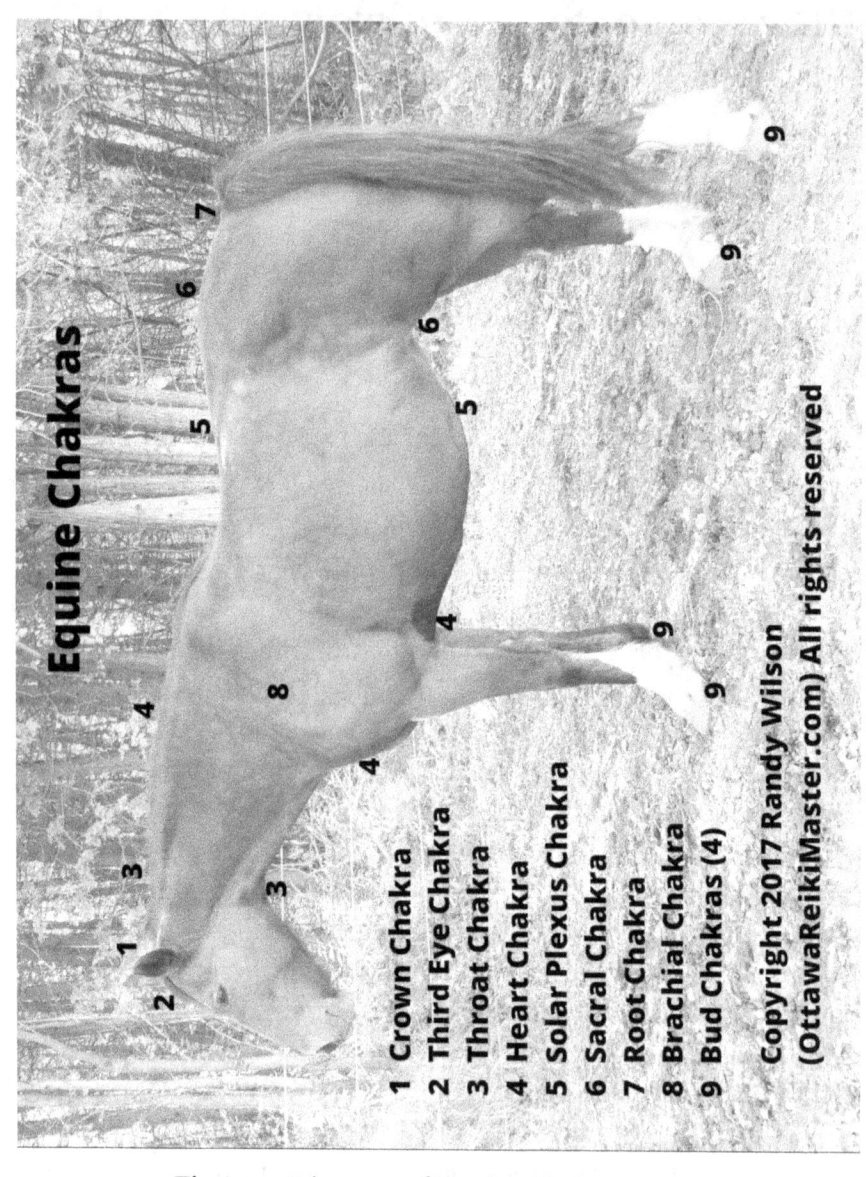

Figure 1: Diagram of Equine chakra positions

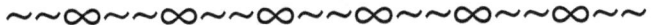

Summary

Everything is energy. Everything is connected. Chakras channel universal energy through your body. They must do it efficiently for you to remain healthy.

PART 2:
Guidelines for Treating Animals

Chapter 4: Energy and Animals

You connect to your clients on an energy level, which means they also connect with you. People usually have a psychological barrier in place to prevent you from knowing all of who they are. They could start sobbing or have any other reaction to a session without knowing why. Or they may know why but will never disclose it, out of guilt, shame, embarrassment, or any other reason. That's perfectly fine. You need to be OK with that. It is not your role to be a counsellor. The Reiki will do what they need it to do for them. You need to accept that the result is totally out of your control. You may never know how you benefited them.

In contrast to people, when you touch animals on an energy level, you usually touch their real selves. Every person and animal is different, of course; there are no hard and fast rules that apply to every living being. But animals will usually present you with the truth: about their lives, about themselves, and about you. They rarely use psychological barriers to shield themselves from unpleasant realities, unless maybe they have been severely traumatized. They carry no guilt, shame, or judgments about who or what they are. You will almost always get the truth; no lies, no deception, no walls, no barriers, no fake facades. It is very real.

When you connect to animals on an energy level, they also touch who you really are. You can't lie to them, nor can you avoid acknowledging how you really feel. They may even know how you are feeling better than you do. So, you need to be in an emotionally stable condition where you can be real with them, because they may be reluctant to accept Reiki from you if you aren't. Apparent lies you may seem to get from them are usually just their difference in perspective. Remember: you don't see the world through their eyes.

There are exceptions, of course, based on an individual animal's background, experiences, or traumas, but it is often true that it can be easier to connect to an animal than a person.

Animal companions are our teachers and mentors. They can help us connect to our spiritual identity and lead us towards understanding who we are. They teach us how to enjoy life, live in the moment, and experience what is happening right now. This is such a wonderful place to be, because this is where life happens, not in our regrets from yesterday or our worries about tomorrow.

We have typically treated animals as possessions; we still buy and sell them. Not so long ago, an animal in Canada had the same legal rights as a piece of furniture. This is changing. For instance, in Quebec, animals are now legally defined as sentient beings and their guardians are obligated to provide proper care for them. This is a significant step towards recognizing animals as sentient beings. Always be aware of this when treating animals: they are sentient souls living this life in animal bodies.

Reiki works the same on animals as it does on humans, and the chakras are basically in the same places. However, how you prepare an animal for a session, offer the Reiki, get his permission, and do the session is very different. Their reactions can vary significantly. When working with animals, you have to be the best you can be. You need to be totally present and emotionally stable. If your thoughts are all over the map (it's called "monkey brain"), the animal will know it and will be reluctant to accept the Reiki. You can't hide your emotions from an animal, even if you can hide them from yourself.

If you are not confident in what you are doing, it will rarely go over well with them. They need to trust you; they will only believe in the energy healing if you do.

Ethics

Informed Consent

Before performing a session, you must get clear consent from the animal's guardian, and also from the animal.

This is about the horse's choice to be in control of his own healing. When you offer Reiki, it is an *offer*. You need to offer it with no agenda, expectation, or demands. Leave behind any need to get the horse to accept it. This can be a challenging shift in your relationship with your own horse. Your horse will typically bend over backward to please you and do whatever you ask of him. That's pleasing behaviour, not free choice.

You need to give him the choice, actual choice. Have you permitted him to say no to you? Many horses get almost no choice in their lives. They are just expected to obey, to bend to our will. Does the horse know there will be no punishment if he declines it? He will feel any anger, disapproval, or disappointment from you if that's how you react. That's not a free choice for him. You must offer the Reiki freely with no conditions attached—that's how you encourage an animal to accept it from you.

Confidentiality

Anything said to you or experienced by a human client must be kept confidential. Even the fact that they came to you for a session is confidential. Do not share your client list or their contact information without their permission. Follow the same guidelines regarding animals and their guardians.

Do I Get a Treat for Accepting This?

NO. Horses learn from every experience they have. I do not offer a horse any food or treats when I am offering him Reiki. No, you can't have a cookie, no you can't have a carrot, no I didn't bring any apples. I don't want any association between Reiki and food, or him thinking treats are a "bribe" for accepting it. It is only the Reiki that I offer. Their choice is to accept it or not.

The Right Way to Approach It

You need to respect the animal and her right to make her own life choices. This prepares both of you to have a clear, honest, and positive exchange of energy and information. The animal must trust your motives in order to be that open with you. If she doesn't believe the exchange is in her best interests, then she will resist the Reiki. She needs to know you have her best interests at heart. You must approach her with love and compassion, as an equal.

Physical issues you find during the session, like tenderness or pain, are usually things you will want or need to share with the animal's guardian, especially if that is why the guardian arranged the session. You cannot diagnose a physical issue; you are just there to report what you find, sense, or are told. It is the guardian's responsibility to take the appropriate action or get the required professional medical treatment. Shamanic principles teach you to always visualize your client as a complete being, not as their injury or disability.[3] Focusing on an injury creates a negative energy frequency. Set an energetic intention that their body or psychological state is already complete and functioning in the way it needs to. Setting that intention will help you to offer them the best treatment possible. Look past their issues and see them as an intact soul in a physical body.

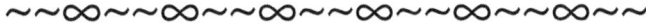

Summary

Animals are sentient beings. They deserve the same respect as a person does. Ask their permission before any physical contact or trying to give them Reiki. They have the right to make their own choices about their bodies and their health. Visualize them as being healthy.

---

[3] The principles of Shamanism mentioned here derive from Core Shamanism, as researched and developed by Michael Harner. To learn more about Core Shamanism, please visit shamanism.org.

PART 3: Doing the Healing Session

Chapter 5: Preparing Yourself for the Session

Preparing Your Mindset

As with everything in life, mindset is everything. One of my favourite sayings is: *"Have a nice day, unless you've made other plans."* You create your own reality. When you wake up in the morning, you typically have already decided how you expect your day to go. You have set the tone for it. If you start your day believing that it will be horrible, then it likely will be. If you start your day expecting it to be positive, then it likely will be. Our lives are not so much shaped by what happens to us as by how we perceive and react to what happens to us.

Likewise, you should approach all your Reiki sessions with a calm and positive attitude, an open mind, and a genuine desire to help. Leave behind any expectations about how the session will progress or what reaction you may or may not get from the horse. You cannot predict the outcome. Trust that the Reiki will do what the horse needs it to do. It is about the horse, not about you. You need to find a reliable way to put your ego aside. Yes, I know, easier said than done. But with practice . . .

The Ego

Ego is your sense of self worth; it defines how you view yourself as an individual. It is part of your unique identity in this three-dimensional existence. Ego can try to convince you that you are superior to other people or animals, which you aren't. It can tell you that your perspective or belief is the only right one. Ego actually has its uses, though. It is a great motivator to push you into action. It also prevents you from being abused and teaches you to avoid unsafe places or situations; it keeps you physically safe. Unfortunately, it can also convince you that nothing is ever good enough. Ego can limit your thinking and convince you that you could never do something perfectly so you should just stop trying.

You need a good balance between acknowledging and accepting your value while still maintaining your humility. Keep striving to improve yourself, but always acknowledge the positive things you have done. Appreciate the healthy boundaries you have set that keep you healthy, physically and emotionally.

Creating boundaries for yourself means letting others know what your limits are. It means having a healthy relationship with yourself where you honour your own feelings, thoughts, and needs. You can't effectively help another person or animal if you aren't healthy yourself. It appears selfish, but your personal well-being always has to come first. You can't give if you have nothing left to give. It's OK to say no, without having to justify it or explain why.

Always approach a horse with your ego in check. Come with the utmost humility and an attitude that you are there to help him, on his terms. You can't tell him you believe you are better than he is, or that you know what he needs or what is best for him. You definitely can't demand that he accept your help. If you approach any animal with that attitude, he likely won't accept Reiki from you.

Rein In Your Energy

You are always projecting energy. Any animal near you can sense your emotions: anxiety, stress, happiness, sadness, excitement, etc.

Animals pick up on every emotional signal from you, so you want to be in a state where you are only vibrating loving and healing energy. If love is the energy coming from your heart, it will calm the animal's fear or anxiety and it will be healing to whatever her needs are. If fear, anger, sadness, guilt, or pity is the energy coming from you, then this will upset her. It will detract from any healing you would like to send.

You need to learn how to rein in your energy and not project your feelings or desires onto an animal. You need to approach animals from a grounded, balanced, peaceful, and respectful state, while not imposing any of your feelings onto them.

Don't approach them demanding that they comply with your wishes or accept physical contact. You need to be a clean slate, open to whatever they want to share with you, physically or emotionally. If you project your needs onto them, they will just mirror them back to you, and you won't be open to hearing what they are trying to tell you.

It's the same with people. When you are talking, you aren't listening. If you have already decided what you expect to see or hear, then you may not see or hear what is actually happening.

An animal has physical boundaries too. If he feels his boundaries are being violated, he could get scared or even aggressive. We all know how an unfamiliar dog will react if we run at him, grab him, and start petting him. Do you like unfamiliar people running up and touching you without your permission? Neither do animals.

Meditation

To enter a horse's world and have her accept the healing, she has to feel comfortable and safe. You need to meet her where she is by being relaxed and in the present moment.

Ideally, you want to be in an alpha brainwave pattern.

What is your brain doing right now? If you are reading this, then you are most likely (or should be) in a beta brainwave pattern. That's where your brain can process logical information and make decisions. Brainwave patterns have frequencies of between 14 and 30 Hz. Frequency is defined as an event within a time frame (one cycle or event per second). One hertz (Hz) is one event per second, like one vibration per second or one foot of distance travelled per second.

Other sources will define these states with slightly different frequency ranges.

Here are the frequency ranges:
Beta = 14–30 Hz.
    A state of concentration, alertness, decision making, and cognitive functioning.
Alpha = 8–13.9 Hz.
    A state of relaxation, presleep, drowsiness,
    meditation, and the beginning of access to
    your unconscious mind (where your intuition lives).

Theta = 4–7.9 Hz.
A state of dreaming sleep (REM), deep meditation, and access to the subconscious mind.

Delta = 0.1–3.9 Hz.
Deep, dreamless sleep.

Beta is the frequency range your brain operates in during most of your waking life. Alpha is where you want to be when treating an animal with Reiki. This is a very calming and attractive mental and emotional state for a horse to find you in. If your mind is wandering all over the past or the future, the horse will be less comfortable around you.

Meditation is a wonderful way to practice putting your mind into an alpha state. It calms your mind and helps limit your internal mental chatter so you can be totally present and also aware of subtle messages you might receive from your equine clients.

Mindfulness meditation is also a great tool for your own spiritual development and mental and emotional balance, even if you do not practice Reiki. It is not as complicated as you might think. All you need is a method that helps you keep your mind in the here and now. One of the simplest ways is to concentrate on your breathing. Your mind is in the current moment when your entire focus is on your breath coming in and going out.

Meditation is not about forcing your mind to do something unnatural to it, like to stop thinking. Our minds think; they always do. We can't control the existence of thoughts, but we can stop them from running into tangents, taking over, and creating little movie scenarios that play on loops in our minds. So, try not to berate yourself for not being able to empty your mind. Rather, focus on quieting it. You want to provide a quiet space for insights and intuition to talk to you. When a thought enters your mind, you simply let it be what it is, then release it and return yourself to the "empty" space in your mind that is between thoughts.

Here are a few meditation strategies:

Concentrate on your breathing going in and out. Ignore all else. When a thought interrupts, just recognize it as a thought, then gently let it go.

When you hear a sound, just recognize that it is a sound, without trying to identify what it is. It is irrelevant to your current intention to create a quiet mind. Then gently let the thought dissipate.

Play the past/future game. When a thought pops into your mind, simply label it as "past" or "future." Then let the thought go. The past is over, you can't do anything about it in the present moment. Any thought focused on the future can wait until your meditation session is over. Unless it is a life-threatening crisis, it can wait until later. This keeps your thoughts in the present moment.

Do any combination of these anytime you need to. Don't get annoyed at your brain for doing what it does, just patiently bring yourself back to the present.

Meditation can be done anywhere and during any activity. You don't have to be in any particular position or play relaxing music. It is about doing anything that will place your mind in the present moment. You can do it while walking, as long as you put all your focus on what is going on around you. Examine the trees and marvel at the new buds. Feel the wind on your face. Listen to the birds chirping outside in the trees. Exercise, with all your focus on what your muscles are doing and how they are feeling. Wash the dishes and focus on the feel of the dish, the water, and the soap on your hands. Anything that causes your brain to be totally present can be considered meditation.

Grounding

I define "grounding" as a state of being totally calm, content, and very connected to and aware of one's physical existence. Being free of anxiety or fear, content to be right where you are and aware of what is happening around you in that moment. When you are grounded, you feel an intuitive connection to the earth and to whatever higher power you believe in, and your personal energy is in tune with your physical existence. I always make sure I am very grounded before I approach a horse. Your first level of Reiki training will teach you how to do this.

One great practice for grounding yourself is to be in bare feet touching the earth. You can be in contact with anything that won't move under your feet the way loose sand does on a beach. Barefoot in the park may be ideal, but indoors in shoes in your office still works. Place your feet flat on whatever surface you have. Get comfortable and balanced, so it doesn't take any effort to maintain the position your body is in. Pay attention to how solid the Earth feels underneath you. You can sense how it is supporting you, holding you up. You can still do this inside a building. The floor is holding you up, while the foundation supports the floor, and the Earth supports the entire building. You are always on a solid surface.

Now, visualize your body connected to the Earth and feel your feet firmly in contact with whatever surface they are on. Concentrate your awareness of the energy in the lower part of your body. Imagine that you are a tree and your legs are the roots. Picture the roots of your tree growing down into the Earth, or through the floor and into the Earth. They dig themselves deeper and deeper. If they find a large rock, they just wrap themselves around it and continue deeper. You can leave them there anchored to an enormous boulder, or let them continue all the way to the centre of the Earth. Now feel how connected you are to the Earth; you and the Earth feel like one entity.

Another example is to connect to or become aware of your earth star chakra. This chakra is about eighteen inches beneath your feet, when they are on the ground. It is your physical link to the Earth. When you recognize your connection to it you recognize your connection to the Earth.

Other daily routines and activities can keep you grounded, like:
- Drinking lots of water; our bodies are mostly water and they need it replenished
- Eating a healthy diet
- Getting regular exercise
- Taking care of your physical and emotional health
- Walking in nature regularly
- Standing still, in contact with a tree
- Being the guardian/caretaker of a pet
- Spending time on activities that you enjoy

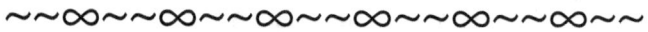

Summary

Learn to place yourself in the best mental and emotional state before offering Reiki to an animal. Treat all animals with respect, as equals. Practice finding ways to leave your ego out of the equation.

Chapter 6: Doing the Session

Now for a complete description of a session. This chapter will cover how I approach sessions, prepare for them, do them, and end them. I will describe what I often see happen and the similarities I find in all sessions. This is not the only way to do a session with an equine client, nor will this method necessarily work best for you or each of your animal clients. You can use it as a guideline of what to expect, what to consider, and what usually works for me. Not that yours (or any future ones of mine) will play out this way. Practice and experience will teach you which of these practices or suggestions is most effective for you or any specific horse. Always pay close attention to his body language and how it changes throughout the session. It will tell you what he likes, what he wants, and what he doesn't.

A Few Reminders

The best results occur after about three sessions, especially if the horse has not experienced this kind of energy healing before. In the first session, he will start getting familiar with the energy pattern, and getting relaxed with you, before deciding to accept it. In general, horses have an innate ability to sense energy. They are also very aware of what they need and what Reiki can do for them. Most horses will settle right into it very well, like a duck to water. Sometimes it takes a little time for a horse to figure out what energy it is sensing and how to use it. Some may take a little longer to decide to accept it.

I suggest that your phone be off, or at least on mute. My family knows when I will be at a stable and I have them text me rather than call me.

If you are going to have a horse led anywhere for the session, it is best if the owner or a stable worker does it. Then you get to do a physical inspection; see how the handler interacts with the horse, how he moves and how he behaves. This gives you a full view of his body movement and a suggestion of any physical issues for you to focus on.

We all have guardian angels, spirit guides, animal guides, and a host of other helpers with us all the time. Ask for their help and guidance with the session, just like you do with your human clients. You need to be calm, balanced and grounded. Trust your intuition and just let the session develop the way it wants to.

A calm and quiet environment works best for the horse and me. It is easier for me to pay attention to what the horse is telling me if I am not carrying on a conversation with someone. Tell the guardian you are happy to explain in advance what they can expect to see happen. Then let them know you will answer any questions they may have after the session. Explain that a quiet environment is more beneficial for the horse to relax into the energy he is receiving. Tell them that to be the most effective you need to focus all your attention on their horse.

You always need to have your equine client's permission, and its human guardian's permission as well. Reassure his guardian that the horse will be OK and that they are welcome to watch. You could also bring them into your Reiki bubble. When I have Reiki energy flowing through me and to a client, the energy emanates all around me for a few feet like a giant bubble. Anyone close enough to be within this bubble will be absorbing some of the Reiki too. If the horse's guardian is close enough to be absorbing some Reiki energy, it will help to relax them too. Tell the guardian that the horse will need an hour or two to rest after the session.

What Will This Be Like for Me?

In a nutshell, doing a Reiki session with a horse will probably feel like any other Reiki session that you have done on a person. You will get all the usual sensations that you get when doing Reiki sessions, including all your usual physical sensations. They can also include any of your usual intuitive, psychic, or emotional messages. You will sense where to go and how long to stay in one particular place, just like you do with people.

It may be a little more challenging in that you have to be aware of your position, balance, and personal safety while you are working on horses. It can be a little more challenging physically. You will be standing on your feet for about an hour. You will also likely hold your arms above your shoulders for long periods. This is common, but isn't a requirement, so if you have a problem doing it see the section below on "Hand Positions."

The other difference is that you will get dirty. Treating horses outside isn't like working in a clean environment like your treatment room. You can't go running for a grooming brush just because the horse decides to lie down and roll over in the mud. You will also be walking through mud, water, snow, droppings, etc. Make sure your boots are suited to whatever environment you will be in.

The Sensations You May Feel

The sensations that you may notice during the session can be any, all, or none of these:
- You may find parts of the horse's body feel hot or freezing cold.
- Any part of your body may get hot or cold (especially your hands).
- You may find your hands tingling.
- You may find your body vibrating or swaying.
- You may feel like a part of the horse's body is pulling your hands towards her, or pushing them away from her. It can feel like the sensations you get when you play with two magnets. If you feel your hands being pushed away, then don't force your hands back to that position.
- You may get random feelings, thoughts, words, or pictures that don't seem to have come from you.
- You may get physical sensations in your body, like a sudden pain in your foot that wasn't there before you started the session. This could suggest a place on the horse you need to address with your hand positions.
- Anything else may happen.

These sensations are all normal. It is also normal for the sensations to vary from client to client, or even from one day to the next with the same client.

Note: Any excessive heat coming from a part of a horse should be pointed out to the guardian and/or addressed by a vet. It can be an indication of a physical issue or injury.

The Best Time and Place for a Session

You can do Reiki anywhere, anytime, but a horse has to feel safe and trust you. Be aware that any environment (inside or outside) with a lot of activity or noise may not be the best place. Noise and activity will catch the horse's attention or take her focus away and could make her a little less willing to accept the Reiki. Ideally, there won't be a bunch of people standing around gawking and chatting either. Sometimes I have found the best place is in the horse's stall, although it carries the biggest risk to your safety. See the section below on safety, for doing this in a stall.

I have found that being tied in cross-ties is not the best option; it tells the horse that she cannot flee. A cross-tie is a strap that connects a horse's halter to the sides of an aisle. One strap goes to a connector on one side of the stable aisle, while another goes to a connector on the other side of the aisle.

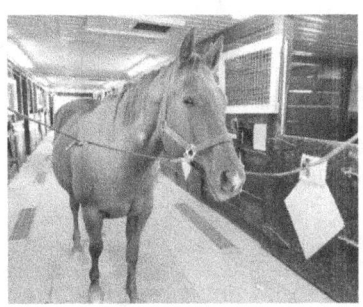

Figure 2: Zip in cross-ties

This is how most horses are held in place while they are being saddled. Since this is supposed to be a relaxing experience and the horse's choice, she needs to know she can walk away from you if she needs to. You don't want her to feel trapped. Everything you can do to minimize the stress for the animal and help her feel safe will always be preferable. I have done many sessions with horses in cross-ties. It definitely works, but it is not my first choice. Cross-ties also come with a greater possibility of distractions in a busy aisle with people walking by, or you needing to unhook one cross-tie to let another horse pass. Anything that disrupts the flow of the session is not ideal.

If you have to tie the horse outside, then I recommend a lead rope and a foot or so of slack. Let the horse move as much as possible while still being safely tied. Use a quick release knot on the rope. A quick release knot is a specific kind of knot that lets the horse pull on it with massive pressure and it will not come undone. The handler can pull on the other end of the rope and it will come freely untied without any effort. This allows for a quick release of the horse in an emergency. A panicked horse can injure himself if he is tied. A horse should only be tied to a solid and immovable object, not to a temporary metal enclosure or a fence board.

It's best to match the time of the session to the horse's schedule, if possible. Early in the morning, horses will want out to run, not stand still in a stall. Just before getting fed, they will be impatient for their food. While they are eating in a stall, they will usually be content to stand still and accept it. It's different again if they are grazing in a pasture. This is why it is essential to arrange the session time with the guardian first.

On the Way to the Stable

When I know I am going to a stable, I unconsciously start my preparation routine. I am already preparing my emotional and mental state for the experience.

I know it will be wonderful just to be around horses, even if nothing else happens or they decline a session. I enter a calm state just knowing I am going. Once I step out of the car, my feet hit the ground and I pull energy up through the Earth to ground me. I accept that whatever is supposed to happen will happen.

Anyone who is at the Reiki second degree will have learned how to do a Reiki session from a distance. You understand how you can make an energy connection to someone who is not in the same room as you. So, I make an energy connection to the animal before

I leave home and I tell him I am coming. I often ask if he is open to receiving some Reiki. This is a very natural thing for me to do, especially with horses I have met before and who already know my energy pattern.

Make the offer again when you get there; sometimes horses change their minds. Be prepared for this because it will happen once in a while. If you get annoyed or disappointed with them for it, they may be less open to it the next time. This is a case of accepting their decision.

This initial distance offer isn't really necessary, but any preparation can help a horse feel more comfortable when you arrive. If he declines it when you get there, just spend time with him to get him used to you and your energy. Give him some time to establish a little trust with you. He is likely to be open to it once he is more familiar with you, especially if you don't push it at him.

If I haven't physically met the equine client prior to arriving at the stable, then it is very helpful to know his or her name, sex, and breed beforehand.

Your Personal Check-In

When you get to the stable, do a personal check-in before you approach the horses.

Our minds think; it's what they do. We all have issues that constantly occupy our thoughts, whether it be about family, money, work, politics, the environment, and so on.

You pull into the parking lot with all this rolling around in your head. Your brain bounces back and forth between these issues and the powerful emotions attached to each of them. The common thread is that none of these relate to anything that is happening in the present moment (except for potential health issues). Everything else is in the past or the future; there is not much you can do about them at this moment.

If you approach a horse while your mind and emotions are scattered, she may not be sure what to expect from you. You need to find effective ways to leave all this at the car. Don't worry about forgetting or losing any of it. It will still be waiting for you when you are done. Don't try pretending that it isn't there either. You can't hide it from a horse, even if you can hide it from yourself.

You need to know what state you are in emotionally and physically. You need to calm all these thoughts, set them aside, be in the moment, be fully present. Use your personal check-in to identify exactly how you are feeling emotionally and physically. Acknowledge these feelings, take ownership of them, then set them aside for later.

Regular meditation is wonderful for this. It can help you train yourself to clear your mind of random or runaway thoughts whenever you need to. It can help get you back to a calm and centred alpha brainwave state quickly. With practice, you can do this in two minutes when you first get to the stable. You can also give yourself a quick five-minute Reiki session to quiet your scattered thoughts and ground yourself.

If you want to communicate with a horse, you need to distinguish between what belongs to you and what belongs to him. You may know the stresses from the day have made you a little impatient or upset. Tell the horse this, and that it is yours and not his. Consciously own how you feel. Then you won't project those emotions onto him, have him mirror them back to you, and think they came from him. This alone will help him be calmer around you. If you are clear with yourself on how you are feeling and how busy your mind is, then you will know what messages the horse is giving you. If an image or word pops into your head, you will know it came from him.

If I get an unexpected or surprising reaction from a horse, I will immediately take a step back, redo my check-in, and re-evaluate my emotional state. Was the reaction his or mine? I may have come in annoyed about something without even realizing it and I need to dissipate this before approaching him again. Was he mirroring how I was feeling? You can't hide your emotions from him, even if you are not consciously aware of your emotions. Always consider what a horse is telling you, because it may be about you and not him. If you still aren't sure, you can ask him whose it is; he'll tell you.

You also need to be aware of how your physical body feels. If you get a sharp pain in your foot, or a sudden headache, you'll know it came from him. You can only believe it if you know for sure that you didn't walk in with a sore foot or a headache.

Clearing the Space for the Session

It's best to begin the session by clearing any unwanted energy from the space where you will treat the horse, whether it be the stable, stall, or even paddock.

All spaces hold energy. You can walk into a room and just sense the feelings and the energy of the people who were there before. It can be a good idea to clear any space in which there had just been an argument or disagreement. Also clear spaces where the energy has been stagnant, like an unused arena or a summer cottage after the winter. It's also a good idea to clear any space that is going to be used for an important event.

There are many ways to clear a space of unwanted energy, and you likely learned at least one way in your Reiki classes. Do whatever process works for you. There is no right way.

Here are a couple of examples:

Example 1.

Step 1. Sit or stand comfortably in the room/space. Breathe in and relax.
Step 2. Set an intention such as "*I ask that Reiki clear this space of any negative energies, entities, or vibrations, and create a space that is tranquil and loving.*"
Step 3. Turn on your Reiki flow. Extend the Reiki in a bubble out from you to encompass the entire room (walls, floor, and ceiling), replacing any negativity with white or golden light. If some areas draw more energy, remain there until you feel it is time to move to the next step.
Step 4. Go to each corner of the room, generate a Reiki ball of energy, and place it there. You will have eight corners and create eight energy balls.
Step 5. Draw a power symbol (CKR) on each door and window.
Step 6. Intend or say "*This room is now filled with love and light, and the spirit of peace dwells here.*"
Step 7. Ground yourself and complete the session.

Example 2.

Step 1. Sit in the middle of the room, draw the power symbol (CKR) on each of your palms, and repeat the name three times.
Step 2. Draw the mental/emotional symbol (SHK) on both of your palms and repeat the name three times.
Step 3. Place one hand on your heart chakra and the other on your solar plexus chakra, and start your energy flow. Keep your hands in this position for about two minutes.

Step 4. Visualize each of these symbols being placed on a wall, while saying, *"I ask that Reiki clear this space of any negative energies, entities, or vibrations. May this room be filled with love and light."*

Step 5. Aim your hands at the wall and send Reiki to it for thirty seconds. Do this for each wall, the floor, the ceiling, and each door and window.

Step 6. Intend or say *"This room is now filled with love and light, and the spirit of peace dwells here."*

Asking Your Guides for Their Help

Once you have cleared the space, you will then start the session like any other, with an invocation asking for divine guidance during the session. You can do this verbally or internally/silently, according to your preference.

Set the intention to allow the healing to take place. Ask for the tools and guidance to help this horse. As with all Reiki sessions, you set your intention for the session to be for the highest good of your client, whether human or animal. Then ask or invite your guardian angels, spirit guides, ascended masters, and any of your other helpers to assist you in the healing session.

We all have helpers from the spirit realm. People use many names for these, like God, Gods, Supreme Being, Source, soul, universal consciousness, higher self, divine beings, guardian angels, spirit and animal guides, ancestors, etc. It doesn't matter who or what you identify with as your divine inspiration. Just know that there is a higher intelligence in the universe and that you are not alone, left to your own devices. There is a wealth of help behind the scenes assisting you in your daily life—all you have to do is ask.

My understanding is that guardian angels will protect you from serious harm. They will never tell you how you must live your life but will always help you in a crisis. Spirit guides will help only if you ask them to. You don't need to know their names or who they are. All you need to do is ask for help and they will help.

None of these divine helpers will ever criticize or judge you, and they will only suggest things that are in your best interests. They will never suggest that you harm yourself or others. Their advice will always be loving, respectful, and supportive. If you get a sense or feeling that some entity is demanding anything of you, attempting to scare you, or suggesting something that just doesn't feel right, then the message you are getting is likely not from a divine helper.

Your helper's messages are subtle, so developing your intuition will help you differentiate between divine help and your ego. Trust your gut; your inner sense of what is right or wrong will tell you. Everyone knows the truth, in that place deep inside themselves: that's your inner compass to what is true and right.

Connecting to helpers is natural and something we can all do. You just have to decide to accept their help, ask them, and be in a calm state, with your mind quiet and receptive. Ask for their help with this healing session, that it be for the highest good of your client. Ask that they assist you in being the clearest and most effective channel for the energy, and to provide you with guidance during the session. Also, ask that they protect you and your personal energy during the session. They will.

Guides will not alarm you or give you something that you are not ready for. They are there to help you with whatever you are ready to accept. They will not propel your life into turmoil, so if they sense resistance or fear in you, they will back off with their message. The more receptive you are, the more you will recognize their messages. The only thing that can block an effective connection to your guides is your fear.

Asking Permission, Offering Reiki

Just as you need to get permission from human clients before beginning a session, you need to get permission from an animal. The animal's guardian is the one ultimately directing her health care needs, so you also need to get their permission.

When you offer Reiki to a horse it is an *offer*. You are allowing her to make her own decision about her healing. You need to respect her decision to accept or decline. Tell her she is free to take as much or as little Reiki as she wants. *This may be the first time someone has ever given her a choice in her life.*

There are many ways to ask a horse's permission. Stand close. Close your eyes and enter a relaxed alpha state. Next, make an energetic intuitive connection and offer the Reiki. Make the offer in your mind and "sense" the answer.

If you use a pendulum, you can set your intention to offer the Reiki, then test the answer you get from the pendulum. You can also use the "sway test." Make the offer in your mind, and you will notice your body swaying either forward and backward or side to side. Forward and backward is a yes, side to side is a no.

Reiki will support an animal's healing on all levels: physical, emotional, mental, and spiritual. You can't know what form that healing will take; you don't even have to know what the animal needs in order for the Reiki to work. Your purpose is just to create a safe space filled with Reiki for her to use in whatever way she chooses. You essentially just start by filling the space with Reiki, and let her come take what she wants. It is not possible to give animals too much, they will only take what they need.

When you offer Reiki to a horse, you are offering it on her terms and have committed to staying until she decides the session is over. Set aside a full hour; sessions are typically somewhere between forty-five and sixty minutes. This is part of the trust relationship that you want to establish with a horse. If she believes you are only going to stay for five minutes, and then leave, she may not accept it at all. Don't panic! You cannot always stay for two or three hours. If it can't be an hour, then set the intention for whatever time frame you have and convey this to her when you make the offer.

Then approach the horse with your mind in a calm alpha state, empty of conscious thoughts, and stand near her in silence for the first two minutes. Start pulling energy from the Earth up through your feet and into your entire body.

Next do a byosen scan. Hover your hands above the horse, and move them slowly along her entire body and notice what sensations you get. You could find areas that are hotter or colder than others. You could notice some areas pulling more energy from you. This gives you the "big picture" of what areas you may need to spend more time on. You learn how to do this in Reiki 1.

When you approach a horse, you have to be receptive to whatever happens, without expectations about what will transpire. You also need to be respectful of the horse's space, and not walk up to it with an air of superiority or an attitude that you know what is best for her. You don't know her history, background, or life purpose.

Let the horse make the first contact. That's your permission to touch her. Otherwise, start at a short distance and wait for a sign that she is OK with your touch.

Start the session if you believe you have permission. Approach her, turn on the flow of Reiki, and place a hand lightly on her brachial chakra. This will usually get you an unmistakable response. If she is open to the Reiki, she will allow this, if not she will move away. If she moves just a foot or so away, stand at a short distance and try "beaming" the Reiki in her direction.

Take your clues from her reaction to decide to continue or not. If she walks to the other side of the paddock, then you may have your answer. Wait for a few minutes, patiently, to see if she comes back. She may need a minute to figure out what just happened (especially if it is her first time), then she may come back for it.

She will decide if she wants it on a particular day. She could decline the session that day and accept it the next. Ten minutes may be what she decides she wants or needs, then she will stop the session. She may want you to continue for an hour or even longer. Younger horses typically want shorter sessions.

A horse may sample the energy, or the intensity of the energy, then decide. She may decide that she wants physical contact or that she would prefer the session from a short distance. If the horse seems to decline the session, it may just be that she wants to decline the physical contact. She may take a little of the energy, then back away to process it, then return for more a few minutes later. If the horse initially backs away from you, it may be to assess your intentions or your sincerity. She could back away to test whether you have the patience and honest intentions to offer it freely and with no expectations. If you are patient and wait, you will probably see the horse come back and accept the Reiki. If she comes close but won't stay in contact, just try providing it from a short distance (a few inches or a foot).

Horses, like all animals, are so sensitive to energy that sometimes they find full contact too overwhelming. From a distance, all the indicators will be there to tell you it is working.

If you are calm and sincere about your intentions, make no demands, and are patient, you will most likely get a yes. I have only ever had one horse completely decline.

Part of getting a horse's permission is helping her understand what is going to happen. If you are taking a horse out of her herd, let her know why. She may be nervous about a stranger taking her somewhere. Reassure her that she is going to a more relaxed or quiet place to receive her session. Walking a horse somewhere lets you see her motion and conformation. That can give you a hint of physical issues to address.

Beginning the Session

Your equine client gave you permission to proceed—now what?

If I haven't already turned my Reiki on, I will generally turn it on now.

Energy travels directly through everything. You don't need to remove a horse blanket or your gloves. If it is warm enough, I prefer to work without gloves. The Reiki penetrates them, but I prefer having my bare hands on the horse. It gives me a more tactile sense of the horse's every muscle twitch, weight shift, or potential upcoming movement.

I start my sessions now by approaching the horse and asking him to take care of me, even if I already know him. I ask him to *"please keep all your feet on the ground when they are near mine,"* and I visualize the horse with all four feet on the ground.

I spend the first few minutes in a relaxed, almost meditative state. I clear my mind, enter an alpha brainwave state, and sense the energy pattern of the horse (essentially just be aware of his presence).

You should approach the horse slowly, and from an angle that he can see you. Stand close, but not in contact. Stay a few feet away so he can get used to you being there, and let him sample your energy. Don't rush right at him and touch him. Some horses will come right to me and make contact, especially if they already know me, but this isn't always the case.

Now offer the first contact with an open hand. Allow him to make the first physical contact, permitting you to touch him. This is one of the first levels of trust you will establish. Most horses get used to having people handle them, without asking for their permission or even giving them the choice. Let the horse touch you first, just like you would with an unfamiliar dog. Also do this with horses you have worked with before; they have moods too and they may not always be open to being handled.

I most often start near the horse's shoulder and offer Reiki at his brachial chakra. This is a good place to start, and the shoulder is one of the safest places to stand near a horse. Touch him lightly on his shoulder, empty your mind of all conscious thought, and just be with him quietly for a few minutes. Remove any expectation of how the session may go. Your auras will merge and you may feel the energy connecting to him.

I will stand near him, watch his breathing pattern, then match my breathing pattern to his. Then I will slow my breathing down, inviting him to match it. He may or may not. Either way is fine.

Talk to the horse with your mind and always visualize the behaviour that you want (not what you don't want). He will often sniff or lick my hand, and I will let him, though I won't allow a horse's teeth in contact with me. When he licks or sniffs my hand, he is testing the energy or the intensity of the energy. He already sensed my energy approaching from about twenty-five feet away. If he is OK with the energy and its intensity, he will stay close and allow me to handle him.

You are there to create a loving and healing space for the horse to choose to walk into—that is your only role. You just need to be you, be calm, and just BE with the horse.

Following the Horse's Lead

In normal handling techniques, you take the lead and just expect the horse to follow, without him being allowed to move you. What comes next can be very challenging. You need to *suspend your normal horse handling techniques and attitudes.* This is not a time to demand compliance, obedience, or ground ownership. It is not a time to reprimand him for his behaviour, unless it is overtly dangerous. Of course, you cannot tolerate any overtly dangerous behaviour, but you need to overlook behaviour quirks. The horse will move you or himself around to get you where he wants/needs you to be. You need to allow this. It's not like he pushes you around but he will make it clear where he wants you, if you are paying attention. You need to allow the horse to be in control of the session. This mutual understanding can take a little while to establish. The horse may have never been permitted to "lead" such a unique dance. This may be a first for him. Once you have worked with a horse for several sessions, he will understand that he has your permission to place you where he wants you. Prepare to be amazed.

Hand Positions

In Reiki 1 you learn the hand positions, that most of them are on the chakra positions, and to spend three minutes on each. You learned them as initial guidelines for how to conduct a session. Now for the "spoiler alert": the chakras are starting points, but they are not absolutes. If you have your Reiki 2, you know that the positions are not critical. You don't need to follow them exactly; rather, just go where your intuition draws you. The Reiki will guide you by indicating which chakras are absorbing the energy and which ones aren't pulling as much energy. If a chakra is pulling more energy, you will feel a stronger energy flow. This indicates that the position needs more Reiki, so you should stay longer on that spot. Recognizing this gets easier with practice.

I usually start at the brachial chakra, then move along each of them, starting with the crown chakra, and stay as long as I feel I need to. Just go where you feel drawn to and the energy will go there. The horse may be too tall for you to reach to the top of his spine, or to hold your arms that high for an hour. You can just move your hands down onto his side, beside the chakra position. It will still work. If he stands still, he is content with it.

Your physical contact should always be positive and direct, not a light touch that would feel like a tickle or a fly. In my experience many horses dislike physical contact on their crown chakra, and often dislike it on their third eye too. I often avoid placing my hands on their crown chakra at all. Sometimes that resistance is just a head-shy horse, so try it from a slight distance. Horses typically need it on their shoulders and their back, through to their dock and their legs. You can also go to the joints on their legs. If a horse can't carry its weight evenly between all four legs, then I won't touch the legs. I will do it from a safe distance of a foot or so.

Sometimes a horse will make a quick jump if you touch a chakra that he doesn't want you on. He could also just bat your hand away with his head. When this happens, I talk to him in my mind. I try to strike a balance between talking to him and listening to him. If he is a little skittish, I will reassure him he is fine and is safe. I will constantly tell him he is free to take whatever Reiki he wants. I reassure him that this is his session and he has my permission to indicate to me where he needs me to be.

If you feel the time is right to move to another position, pay attention to the horse's behaviour. He may accept the move or tell you to go back to where you were. He may tell you to move, he will move himself, or he will move you to get you where he wants you. This is incredible to experience! *Not all horses will want physical contact.* He may show you that he wants it from a short distance. If he moves just out of contact, allow it, and just stay about a foot away. If he isn't running away, then you need to trust that it is working, even if it isn't going the way you expect.

The energy may overwhelm the horse in a particular area and he will need your hands moved elsewhere. You will eventually get more experience reading the body language of horses and interpreting what they are telling you.

Once you can follow their instructions, you will recognize that they are telling you exactly where they want you. If a horse moves forward or backward by a foot while you have your hands on him, the natural tendency would be to go with him, *but don't*. Just keep your body and hands exactly where they are. You will probably find that he has moved his body to get your hands to where he wants them. You may begin with your hands on his solar plexus chakra and then find that you are now on his sacral chakra. He just placed you there! Then he is standing perfectly still again once he put you where he wanted you. Horses become very adept at doing this. I have had horses spin themselves completely around in a stall to get me to the other side of them. It doesn't get much clearer than that!

One horse I work with isn't as clear with his instructions. I seem to get conflicting body language clues from him and have to keep asking him what he wants. It's probably because I just haven't learned how to read him very well yet. I am sure he is telling me, and I'm just not listening carefully enough. If this happens to you, then pay closer attention to all the body clues you are getting. You are in the right place if he stands still. He may even want you on that one spot for the entire session, and that's OK. It is his session and he is directing it. You are there to provide what he needs. I think I still occasionally let my ego get in the way and go where I want to go. I try to stay in my intuitive state, where this won't happen.

As with any session, the Reiki and your intuition will tell you where to go. If the horse isn't happy with you there, he will move away slightly. It will be a very subtle shift in position, so you have to be paying attention. Sometimes a look over his shoulder at you could say:

"*Why are you still on that spot? I asked you to move over there. Aren't you listening?*" Unfortunately, it could also say: "*Where did you go? I need you back where you were!*"

You may notice more or less energy being pulled from you at various positions. You may notice hotter or colder areas. All the same clues you get with people will show where you need to place your hands.

There's one thing to know about physical injuries. Any open wound or broken bone is not a place to put your hands. Bones have to be properly set before they start healing. That applies to people too. The intensity of Reiki in direct contact with an injury is usually not welcome by animals. Instead, do it from a distance. You could also place your hands on the nearest chakra point to the injury, or on the ones both above and below it.

The figures that follow demonstrate hands placed on each of the chakra positions.

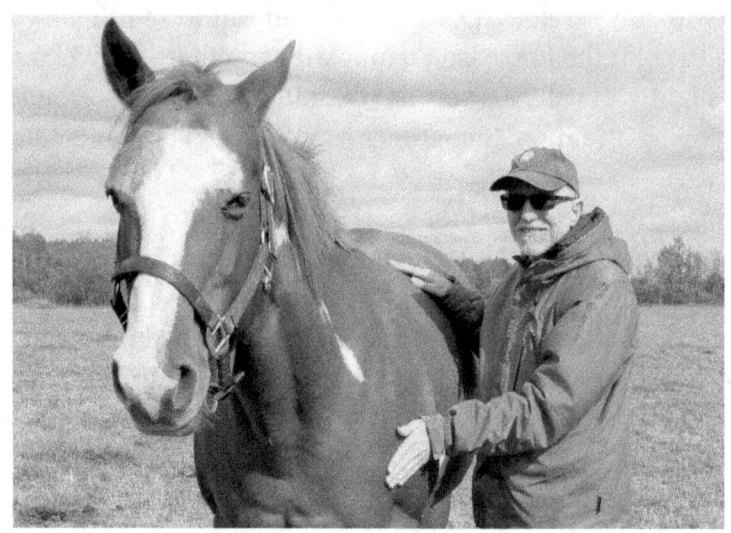

Figure 3: Starting point at brachial chakra

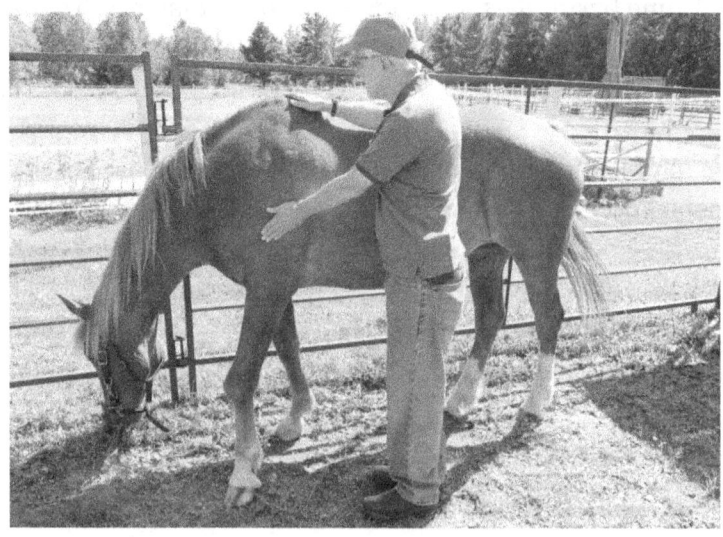

Figure 4: Starting point at brachial and heart chakras.

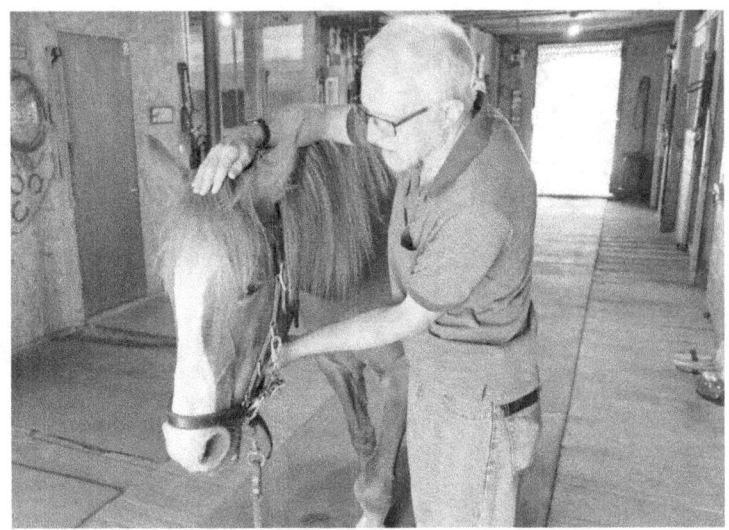

Figure 5: Crown and throat chakras

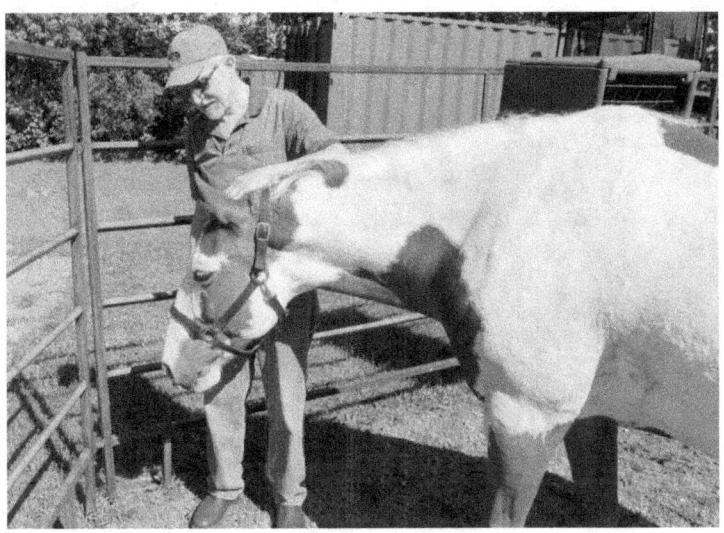

Figure 6: Crown chakra

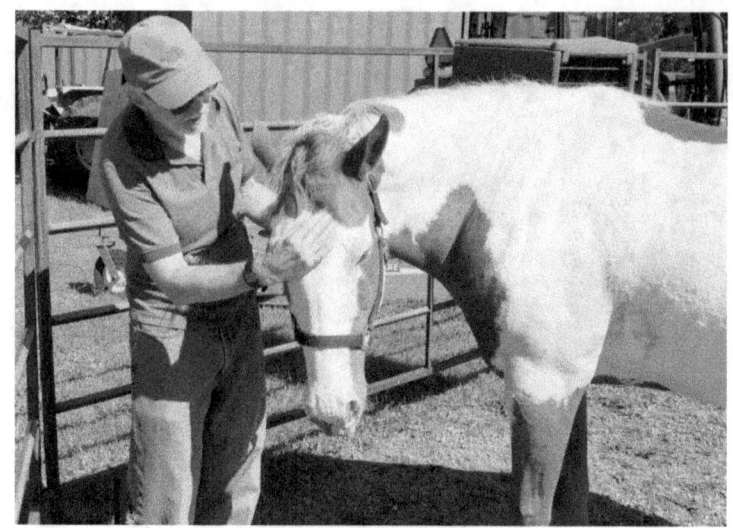

Figure 7: Third eye chakra

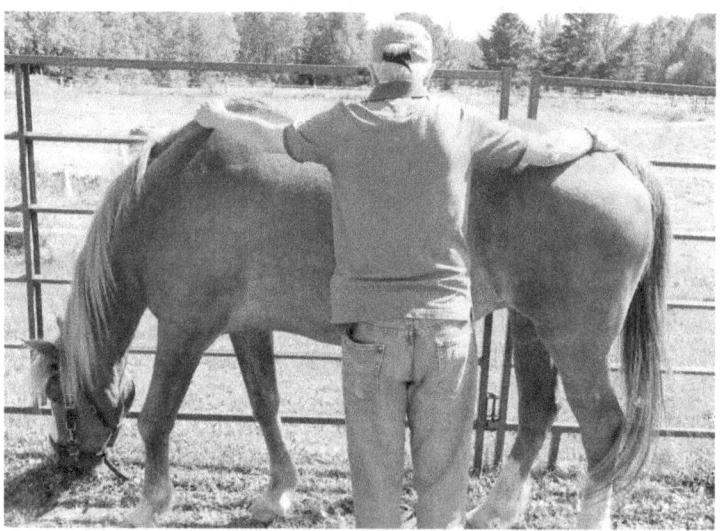

Figure 8: Encompassing heart to root chakras

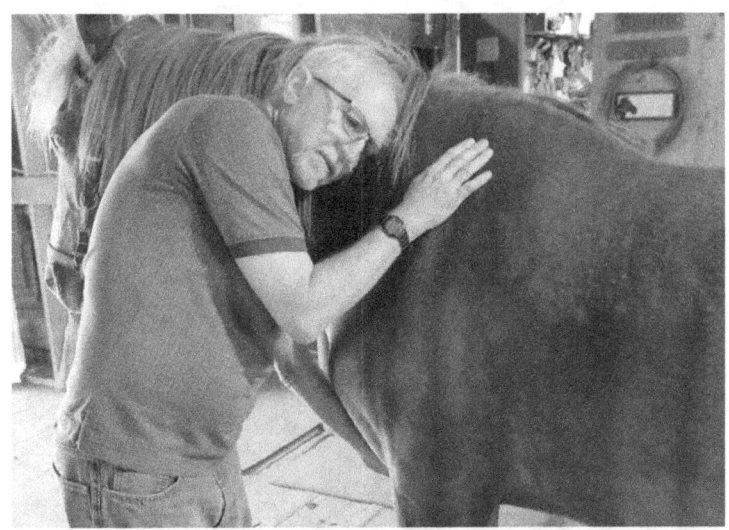

Figure 9: Heart chakra

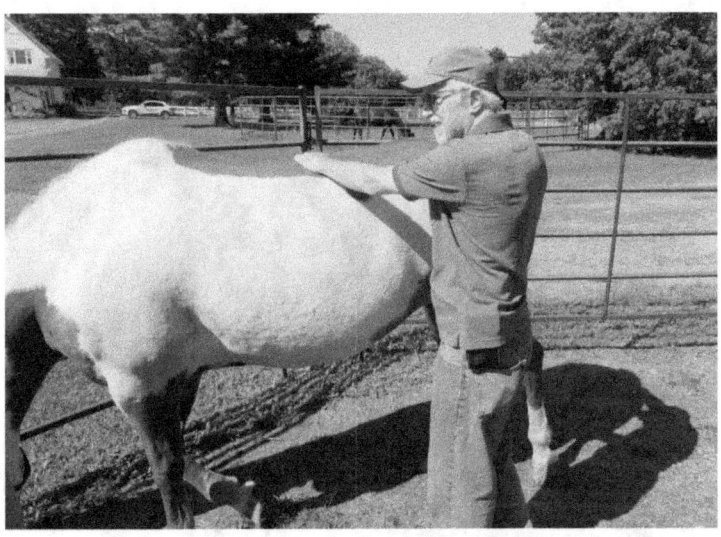

Figure 10: Solar plexus chakra

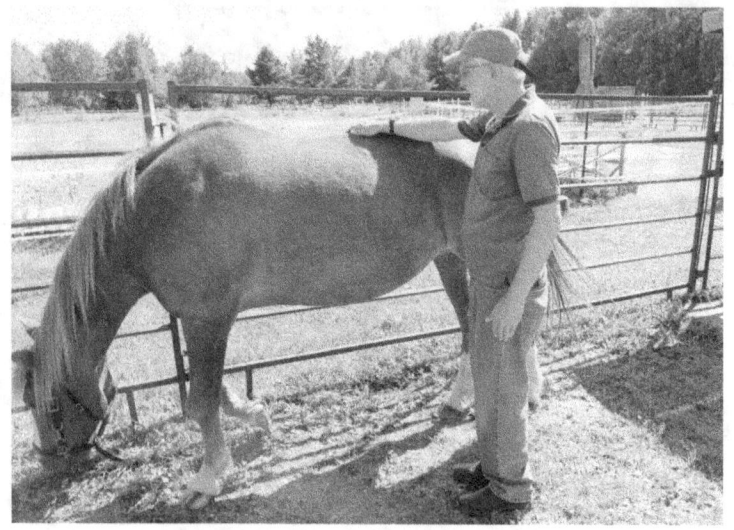

Figure 11: Solar plexus chakra

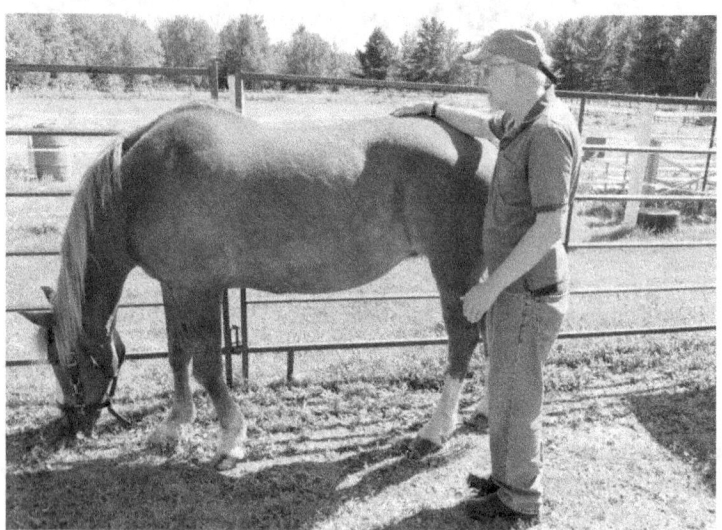

Figure 12: Sacral chakra

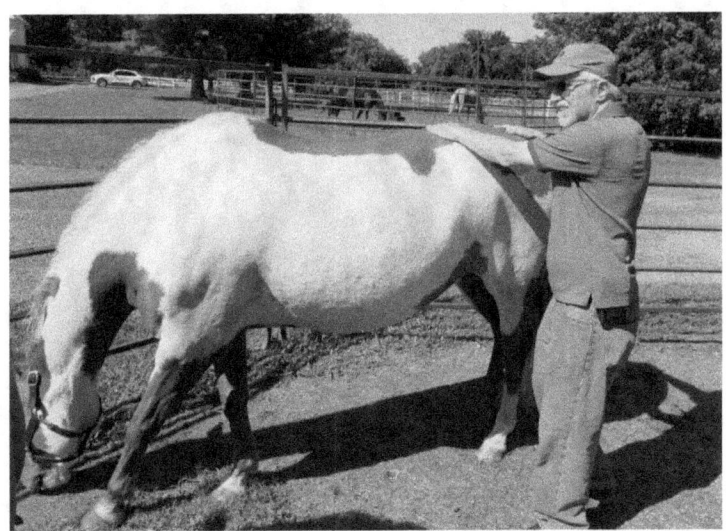

Figure 13: Sacral and root chakras

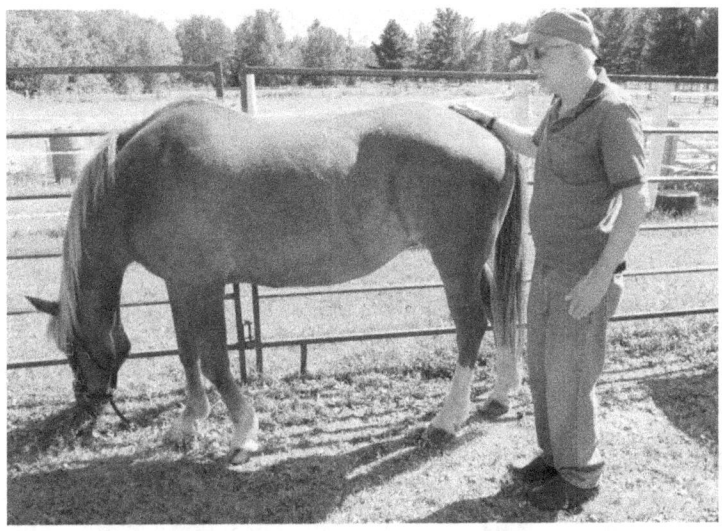

Figure 14: Root chakra

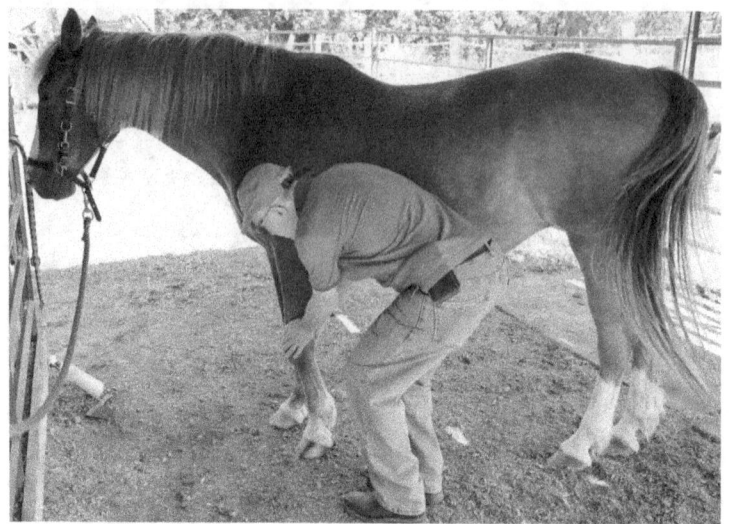
Figure 15: Working on a swollen knee

What Reactions You Might See

You may get no sign at all that it is working, and that's fine. Trust that the Reiki is working and that it is doing what is in the best interests of the horse. This can be a challenge when you are just starting. Trust the Reiki.

Here are some indicators that the horse may or may not give you when he is receiving and processing energy.

You will normally always see their breathing rate change.

You may see any, all, or none of these indicators:
- Any normal sign that he is relaxed
- Muscle twitching
- Licking and chewing, lips quivering

- Lowered head, below the poll
- Head lowering to the ground, bobbing back up, then lowering to the ground again
- Gurgling stomach
- Urination or bowel movements
- Snorting, yawning, or sighing
- Eyes soft or glazed over
- Eyes partially or totally closed
- Falling asleep
- Lying down for a nap during or after the session
- Head shaking, to shake off excess energy
- Pawing at the ground
- Standing motionless
- Moving away for a short time, then coming back
- Moving just into or out of contact with you
- Moving his head around to look at you
- Leaning into you to stay in contact
- Males will often drop their penis if they feel a strong "heart" connection (it is not sexual)
- Bucking, jumping, or running away when he first feels the energy
- Exploding into a flurry of motion
- Kicking at the air (he can sense the energy and may think something is there)

The following figures show you what totally relaxed horses can look like when they are in my Reiki bubble.

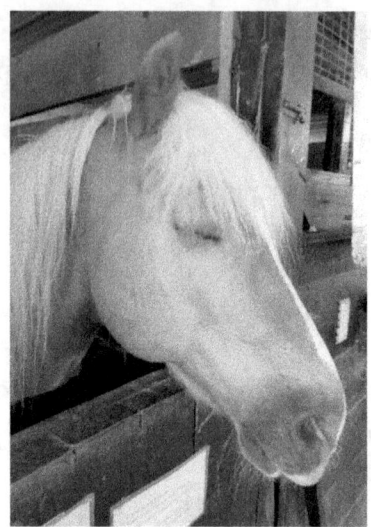

Figure 16: Monty asleep

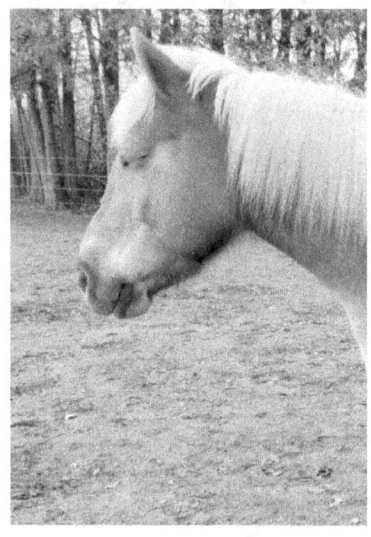

Figure 17: Kasper asleep

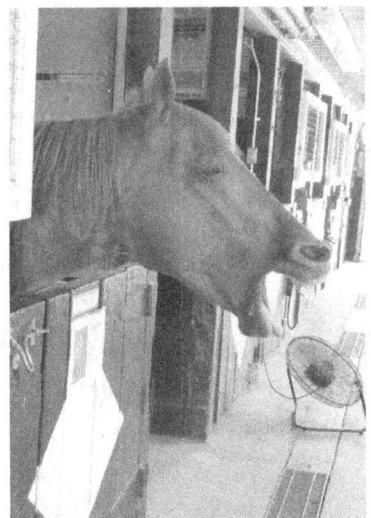

Figure: 18 Chica yawning

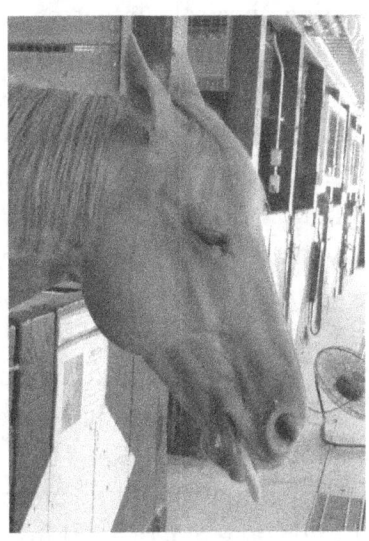

Figure 19: Chica with tongue hanging out

Although I have seen horses pee during a session, it seems more usual for them not to. They often wait until the session is over. During a session in a stall, they will move away from you to leave droppings, or spin around and leave them in a corner. If you are not in a stall, they may (and often do) walk away from you first. If they walk away and leave droppings, they will probably come right back to continue the session. This is not the same as them walking away to tell you the session is over. A Reiki session with a horse is an exercise in patience. If he isn't running away from you, then he is content with it and you need to trust that it is working, even if it isn't going the way you expect.

Wait, That's Just Way Too Intense!

If the horse is resisting physical contact, she may find the energy too intense and would prefer to receive it from a little farther away.

Your other option is to turn down the intensity of the Reiki energy that you are channelling (generating).

"Hey, wait just a minute there, what are you talking about? I thought Reiki was either on or off."

OK, I'll explain. If you are at the Reiki first degree, then this may be a new concept for you. At that level, you are usually thinking about turning it on and worrying about whether it really is on.

In my Master class, I learned how to adjust the intensity of the energy. You do this with intention, just like you do when you turn your Reiki energy on. Someone at the Reiki first degree should be capable of doing this, too. It may be a little more difficult, or just take extra awareness and some practice. I think the intensity, consistency, and frequency range of the energy you can channel at the Master Level lends itself to a greater range of adjustment. At the first degree, the difference between your lowest and highest frequency level may be too subtle, or the consistency may fluctuate too much, so it may not lend itself easily to that kind of variance.

So, here's your homework. Practice this visualization and you'll get it.

Set your intention to adjust the intensity. Calm your mind, sense the Reiki energy flowing through you. Imagine or visualize it flowing through your hands in waves of energy. Now picture the frequency or intensity being at 100 percent of what you can generate. Imagine a volume control knob on each palm. Slowly use your other hand to adjust it to something at a lower intensity. Forget about weird numbers; set levels to a couple simple values, like 25, 50, and 75 percent. At first, just try setting it to 50 percent. Now imagine the Reiki energy matching the level that you set it to. Do this on both palms and believe the intensity has decreased.

With practice, you will be able to do this just by simply deciding you want it to happen. Don't get hung up on seeing your volume control knob move; energy work is all about your intention, and not related to any specific hand gesture.

There is a horse named Howard who I have treated regularly. His decision about wanting physical contact changed daily. Some days he wanted full contact, and on other days he didn't. Sometimes I needed to just spend time with him with my Reiki turned off. After about ten minutes I would turn it on to 25 percent, offer it, and wait for a sign that he was OK with it. If he accepted it, then I would turn it up to 50 percent and leave it there for five or ten minutes. If he was still OK with that, then I could usually turn it up to 100 percent and complete the session. This process worked well for this horse. Every horse is different. Always assess the messages you are getting; he is telling you exactly what he wants and needs.

Animals are extremely sensitive to energy patterns, more so than people are. I have never found a reason to turn down the intensity with a person—they always get 100 percent of the intensity of my Reiki.

But I Don't Want You There

I had an occasion early in my practice when my mind wandered and I wasn't paying enough attention to recognize a sign. I had one hand on Howard's brachial chakra and one on the top of his neck above his heart chakra. I had been there for five or ten minutes and he stayed still, so I thought everything was just fine. Out of the blue, he flipped his head around and batted my hand right off his body. He hit me hard enough to cause pain and a bruise. He startled me and I jumped, which of course made him jump.

I quickly told him he was fine and safe, and that everything was OK. Then I told him I was sorry that I missed the cue and thanked him for telling me he needed me to move.

Learn to take these as teaching moments and thank the horse for them. You need to find a way within yourself to allow these moments to happen without getting angry, blaming him, or chastising him. He gave you a sign that you missed. He needs to direct his session without you getting upset with him for it. You need to allow him to tell you what he needs without worrying about how you will react. Every session I do teaches me something. That's also why I make notes right after every session.

Heart to Heart

A horse may resist letting you place your hand on her heart chakra in the middle of her chest. This is a very intimate connection that she may not allow. Horses need to get to know you and develop some trust before they accept you there. They will usually be happy with you at their heart chakra position on the top of their neck on the withers. The middle of their chest is often the last place I approach in a session. Once they are comfortable with me and the energy, they may allow it, and often do. Remember that this is about the horse, not you, so don't insist on any specific hand placement. Do only what the horse is comfortable with.

When a horse allows this and truly connects with you on this level, you'll know it when it happens. You will experience a deep sense of love and acceptance, and feel as though you and the horse just became one being. Some of these feelings can happen in a regular session, but a "heart to heart" connection with a horse is extremely intense! You could be surprised and completely overwhelmed. If there is ever a time in an Equine Reiki session that will bring you to tears, this is it. Don't push this to make it happen or you'll just scare the horse away from allowing it. It has to just happen on its own. Then break out the Kleenex.

A Crying Horse

During one session, as I approached a horse on stall rest, I gazed into his eyes and they seemed distant, like he wasn't totally present. I felt an overwhelming sadness well up deep inside me. Once the horse saw me, he immediately started struggling to catch his breath. His heart was racing as he gasped air in and out rapidly.

He was trying, unsuccessfully, to stifle a major outburst while his chest heaved. This continued for a couple of minutes. As the gasps got slightly longer, they took on a higher pitch on each inhale and their timing got more erratic. Eventually the intervals started getting longer and his chest stopped pounding. Then came the slower, deeper breathes as a calmness started to waft over him and he returned to a relaxed state.

I was both overwhelmed and humbled to witness a horse be that vulnerable and honest with me. A horse's behaviour tells you how he feels, but most people don't actually feel it too.

Through it all I just stood outside his stall door, closed my eyes, and stayed in the moment. I really believed I was hearing someone struggle to stifle a major crying fit. You know what I'm talking about, how this sounds and feels; you've probably done it yourself. For us, I think we would all be better off just allowing ourselves to break down into a sobbing fit instead of hiding it. Most people aren't capable of standing by and watching someone cry, they want to jump right in and "fix" it. However, I just stayed in the moment with him and let him be what he needed to be. I even think we have a closer relationship now.

I know a lot of research says horses can't cry, but their evidence refers to a horse's inability to shed tears. Crying is more than just tears.

Treating Horses in a Stall

Treating a horse in a stall can often be the easiest location. It's ideal if the stable is quiet, without a lot of talking or activity. When in a stall, there are often no other horses in view or distractions that could catch the equine client's attention. There is also nowhere for the horse to go, so she will stand more still. Most stalls have enough room for horses to move away from you when they need to.

I find it's ideal in the late afternoon or early evening when most of the guardians or students have left for the day. It doesn't get much better than being alone with a horse in a stall in a quiet stable.

Be aware that this can also be the riskiest, most dangerous place to be. It is an enclosed space. You can't run or push the horse away from you to get more distance. You can also be squashed against a wall if she spins unexpectedly. Regular workers have had that happen to them just being in there for a few minutes. You can assume that to stay in a stall for an hour comes with even more risk. For more information, see the section below on "Safety, in a horse's stall."

Treating Horses Tied to a Hitching Post

A hitching post can be a common place to conduct a session. The stable owner may not be comfortable with you in a pasture or paddock with other horses. They may allow it but require you to wear a helmet. It may be an insurance issue for some stables. They may be OK with you in a stall only if they have sliding doors that can be left unlocked so you can get out quickly; or with a rope across a fully open door, and you stay at the door.

If a horse is tied to a hitching post, it should be in a place away from a barn door or busy traffic area. Try to give her a little slack on the lead rope, so she has some ability to move about. This will give you full access to all sides of her. She will still be able to move around enough to get out of physical contact with you if she wants to. Still, you will need to be very aware of the horse's body movements. She can't just walk away to end the session. She also can't move her head out of contact with you if she doesn't want contact there.

Use a quick release knot to tie the lead rope. Only tie it to an immovable object, like a buried fence post. Do not tie it to the cross board of a fence or to any temporary fencing.

Some stables may use dedicated halters or lead ropes for their horses. You may be going out to the herd to offer the Reiki then come back in to the barn to get the halter for the horse that accepted. With your Reiki 2 you can connect to each of them from outside the paddock, identify the horse who wants it, then go in with her halter. If you have Reiki 2, you can also do a byosen scan on each of them from a distance to identify which one to offer the session to. This may not always work because sometimes they all want it at once, as I discuss in the chapter "Herd Dynamics."

Treating Horses in a Sand Ring, Arena, or Dry Pen

A sand ring, arena, or dry pen can be one of the best places to perform a session since the horse can't wander around and graze. Her body movements and signals can be easier to interpret since she likely will be moving less.

When you are outside, you may have to adjust your expectations about the sensations you will get. You may not feel any energy transfer from your hands. The wind may mask the sensation of the energy moving between your hands and your client. Many Reiki practitioners use these sensations as a sign of where to place their hands and where the energy is being pulled from. Some even question whether the Reiki is working if they don't feel the sensations. You have to trust that it is working.

You may want to clear the energy in an arena just like you clear any room you work in. Arenas can carry residual energy from whoever was in there previously. It could have been a very frustrated horse and rider from a lesson that didn't go as successfully as either of them had hoped. It could just be very stale and trapped energy if nobody has been in there lately. Clearing the energy before your session will allow the Reiki to be as effective as possible for your client.

If you put a horse into an arena she is not normally in, it will be an unfamiliar environment for her. Know that it may take her a little extra time to get comfortable there. If the arena is full of jumps and she doesn't like jumps, or if it is full of unfamiliar objects or clutter, these objects could add stress.

Horses are curious souls. If you give them anything that they can consider a toy to play with, they will play. They may be more interested in playing with their newfound toys than accepting the Reiki. You can isolate them from these distractions by running some posts and a rope across part of the arena, so they are in their own isolated space. The key is to accommodate each horse by finding what works best for them in each situation.

Treating Horses in a Pasture

This can be a little more challenging, if only to your confidence level. I find it much easier to interpret a horse's movements if they are in a stall, arena, or a dry pen/paddock. The horse will stand more still if she isn't grazing for food. When a horse stands motionless or repositions herself to get me where she wants me, then I know she is happy. In a pasture, horses constantly move while they graze. *"Did they just move to get you to change positions, to get to a greener patch of grass, or to get away from you to end the session?"* They often show the end of a session by moving away or eating or drinking, but that just doesn't apply if they are moving and eating the entire time. With practice, you will get used to following their movements and being aware of the other clues they give you.

If the horse is a little more skittish, it may be beneficial to have the guardian or a stable worker there with a lead rope on the horse.

Treating Horses Outside, with Others Nearby

You need to come to an understanding with the guardian as to which horse you will be treating. They may need assurance that the horse they asked you to treat is getting the Reiki. But if there are other horses in the pasture, which one gets it? The answer is whichever one you focus on and intend to give it to . . . oh, and any other horse nearby.

If the guardian wants guarantees, then you may need to isolate the horse from the rest of the herd. This is not necessary, but be sure the guardian understands that. As long as the horse is getting your direct attention, she is getting the full benefit of the Reiki, even if she is sharing it with the herd.

The key is to focus your full attention and your intuition on the horse you are treating. This is a skill that can only come with practice. You will want to sense everything the horse is feeling and where she wants your hands or the energy to go. You need to be aware of whatever messages she is giving you. This can't happen as easily if others are piggybacking off the energy by being in contact with the horse you are treating. Yours would get what she needs, but you may miss some signals that you would want to be aware of.

Any horse in contact with you or the horse you are working on, or within a few feet of either of you, will absorb some Reiki. As long as another horse isn't trying to push your client away to get some energy, then it's all good.

Reiki is limitless, there's always plenty to go around. Let the guardian know that a horse sharing it with the herd does not diminish the amount available to the client. The horse may share it, or not. The others may jockey for position to get close to the energy. Their antics can be hilarious but also maybe a little distracting for you. See also the chapter on "Herd Dynamics and Reiki."

Time for Another Horse

Start the entire process *from the beginning* before you approach another horse to offer him a full session. Wash your hands, ground and centre yourself, ask your guides for help, and ask permission of the horse.

You may be in a pasture offering Reiki to many horses at once. You can't easily leave and come back every time you approach another horse, so just go from one horse to the next. One option is to disconnect your energy from one horse when you approach another, but they will usually all be too close together for that.

In such an environment, the session flows naturally from one horse to the other. When they are in a herd, they just seem to understand that they are sharing your focus. You will probably find them casually come into and out of your Reiki bubble. Although for you it may feel very different from a one-on-one session, the horses will still benefit from the Reiki.

When to End a Session

You don't end a session with an animal according to a specific duration. A session ends *when the horse tells you it is over*. Usually, the horse will end the session after forty-five to sixty minutes, so plan on being there for at least an hour. That's the agreement you made when you offered it.

Younger horses typically prefer shorter sessions. The session could be as short as ten or fifteen minutes. When the session is over you will usually know: the horse will make it very clear when he has had enough.

Signs that a horse wants to end the session:
- He might get more animated and start moving around more
- He could shift his body slightly away from you every time you touch him
- He might walk away or back away from you
- He could push you away
- He might start eating or drinking
- You may also feel or experience signals within your own body, indicating that the session is complete.
- You could feel an energy shift
- Your hands will stop channelling energy
- You could sense a subtle "disconnection," like he is not there anymore
- You won't feel a need to go anywhere else on his body
- You could experience the "pendulum effect"
- Any indicator you would get with your human clients
- Your intuition will tell you

If the horse's stall is big enough for him to turn around in, he can still get away from you. He can create distance from you by backing away into the far wall or corner, out of contact. I have had horses walk a circle around me to the other side of the stall behind me. Then I was facing an empty wall, with my back to the horse. I think that's pretty clear.

If you are unsure of the signals that the horse is giving you, you can ask him if he has had enough. You could also experience the "pendulum effect" (or sway test) that you may have used when you first offered him the Reiki. Ask the horse if he is ready to end the session. Then stand still and find your body swaying back and forth. This is very subtle, so you have to be paying close attention to notice. Forward and backward is a yes, side to side is a no. You can also use this technique for any question you want to ask.

Your intuition that serves you so well when working with human clients will also tell you when the session is over with equine clients. With practice you will know intuitively.

How to End a session

So you believe the session is over. Now what? Dart away in a flash! Get away from there as fast as you can!

No, please do not do that. You need to complete the session in a calm and gentle way. Don't just go from full-on Reiki to instant physical and energetic disconnection. It's too abrupt.

What you'll want to do is sweep the horse's aura completely from her head to her root and down the back of her legs. Then, brush the energy off your hands in a quick swipe across your palms a few times. Do it a few feet away from the horse, not under her. This is called a "bladder sweep." It will release any excess energy, just as it does for your human clients. Do this on both sides of the horse. Then go to her head and thank her for accepting the Reiki from you. Then step away.

If the horse is in a pasture or paddock, she may have walked away from you to end the session. When this happens, I don't attempt to go back to do a bladder sweep. If she has had enough, she won't let me that close anyway, she will just walk away again. This is where Reiki 2 ability comes in. I do an energy sweep from a distance and thank her for the session, from a distance.

Now ground yourself. Ask Reiki or your guides and masters for help to disconnect the energy. Return all energy to the horse that belongs to her. Return to the Earth any energy that does not belong to the horse. Clear all energy from your aura that isn't yours. Have all energy that does not belong to you returned to whoever it belongs to, or returned to the Earth.

Next, disconnect the energy connection between you and the horse. I typically use a power symbol (CKR) to do this, as an on/off signal to myself to change my focus and intent into or out of a Reiki session.

You can then provide the horse with food and water, and drink a large glass of water yourself.

Remind the guardian that the horse needs an hour or two to rest after the session, to process and integrate the energy she received. This is not a time to make her do any physical activity. She may be sleepy or dopey, so she may lie down and have a nap. Reiki keeps working even after the session is over, so I won't give two sessions to a horse on the same day.

Remind Me of What Just Happened

Immediately after every session, I make some quick notes before I leave the stable, while everything is still fresh in my mind. Record them immediately; it is too easy to forget those subtle details. It only takes a few minutes and a few sentences to serve as a reminder for when I get home, when I add a more detailed description. I describe what happened, what I did, what the horse did, what I sensed, what I learned, what worked, and what didn't work. I describe what reactions I got from the horse and, just as importantly, what he and I were doing when it happened. What the horse teaches me during the session is also well worth noting. Most of the content for this book came from my session notes and my own experiences.

Distance Sessions

Once you have your Reiki second degree, you will know how to connect to the energy pattern of someone at a distance and offer them a Reiki session. You use the distance symbol (HSZSN) for this. This works just as effectively as a hands-on session in person.

To conduct a distance session, all you need is a way to identify the specific person or animal that you want to send the session to. There are a number of ways to do this. For me, one of the simplest ways is to have a photograph with only them in it. With an animal it's best if I can clearly see his or her eyes. Any way that you can identify a specific person or animal works. For example, you can identify them by having their name and/or address. You can also identify them by their association to someone else: a friend's father or the name of the animal's guardian. That is enough, as long as you are specific about who.

You won't have the person or animal in front of you, so there are some different methods for doing the session. You can look at the photo or their name and address on paper as you do the session. Visualize the equine client in front of you, or visualize the human client on your table, and simply tell the Reiki to go to them. As you do the session you can visualize your hand placements. You will even feel the energy transfer through your hands as if the client was right there with you. Another option is to use a surrogate to represent the client. A teddy bear works well.

You can also use this ability to connect to the horse you intend to visit in person. You can make the offer and know if the horse is receptive to accepting it before you leave for the stables. Remember that a horse can change his mind. Even if you get a yes before you leave home, he could change his mind before you get there. I find this rarely happens. I also find horses can say no and when I get there, they are open to it. Now, I usually just connect to them and tell them I am coming; I set the scene and my intention to help them.

Distance sessions do not have to be out of the country, out of the city, or even out of sight. With your Reiki first degree, you are usually in contact with or reasonably close to your client. With your second degree, you can perform a session from a short distance, such as from outside their stall, the other side of a fence, or from halfway across a paddock. Do this if it isn't safe to be in their stall, or if you have a nervous, aggressive, or dangerous horse that you can't safely get close to.

Follow the same process that you do for a hands-on session. Offer the Reiki and accept the horse's answer. Anything you can do in close contact you can do from a distance (with Reiki 2). You can also do a bladder sweep and disconnect yourself energetically at the end of a session, all from a distance.

Doing a session from a distance can be easier. You can do it in the comfort of your home, in a nice relaxed atmosphere, with no distractions. You have no safety issues to be concerned about, like being stepped on or knocked over. You don't get distracted by crazy antics; they can be hilarious, but they can affect your focus and concentration. You don't have other horses intruding or fighting over the Reiki. You don't have to watch the entire herd for indications that your horse or the others may scatter. There are no weather issues like hot sun, pouring rain, high winds, freezing cold, wading through mud, or bugs biting you or the horse. As you can see, having your Reiki second degree comes with endless benefits.

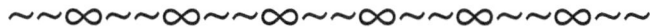

Summary

This is the meat of the book. Have fun with it. Practice. You don't have to memorize all these steps. There is a checklist coming later.

Chapter 7: Ways to Enhance a Session

Chakra Balancing

Another form of energy healing is chakra balancing. Chakra balancing goes hand-in-hand with Reiki, since a session typically balances chakras at the same time. It will happen as a by-product of the session or you can specifically do it if you see a need.

You will often find that when you sense energy being pulled from your hands that it happens at a chakra position. Chakras should all spin freely, in the same direction, and with the same intensity. They will feel like energy vortexes that resemble the cone of a tornado swirl. When you place your hand over a chakra, you can sense the intensity and direction of the energy.

There are many ways to test chakras to be sure of their movement. A pendulum dangled over a chakra will show you its direction and how wide the swing is. You can also place one hand on a chakra point and hold the pendulum in your other hand. The direction, speed, and diameter of the chakras should all match. If you find one not moving, or moving very little, that's one place for your hands to spend time on. Then retest it to see the change.

A pendulum does not have to be store-bought. I wear crystals on chains, so I always have one available. A pendulum just has to be something with a weighted end that is balanced so it can spin consistently.

You can balance one chakra at a time as you move down the body. Placing your hand over a chakra with your Reiki running will help balance it. Once you have done them all, you might go back to the first one and find it is unbalanced again. It's not always a case of doing them all once and being done. If one is off, or not the same as the others, just do it again.

You can do two at a time, with one helping the one beside it. One chakra may still be really unbalanced. You can adjust that one by balancing the one on either side of it at the same time. Once you think you are done, go back to the first and check each one again. I don't always go through this process because I find Reiki typically balances them all by the time I finish the session.

You can also balance them with a pendulum. Holding the pendulum over the chakra will get it rotating. Keep the pendulum there until it rotates clockwise and has a consistent amount of swing over each chakra.

I can also coax chakras into spinning using Reiki. I use my hand, rotating at the wrist, to start a swirl of clockwise energy. The chakra will match my movement and start rotating. I increase the speed until I get a six-inch diameter spin.

You can accomplish this in other ways, like Shamanic healing techniques, meditation, crystals, and so on.

If the horse's guardian informs you of a specific health issue, then you would specifically balance the chakras related to that part of the horse's anatomy or the organs involved.

Recently a farrier told me he thought the horse I was about to approach had an issue with his back leg. The horse told me his pain level was a three. He wasn't in his usual stance. He was shuffling his balance back and forth between his back legs uncharacteristically. Sometimes he had his legs in a square, balanced stance. Sometimes he had one foot in the middle of his body in a triangle. This was very unusual for him. When he lifted his right leg, he kept it in the air for about twenty seconds before he put it back down. I had never seen him do that before. I approached his right stifle and attempted to touch it. When I made contact, he instantly leaped a foot sideways. If his guardian had seen it, she would have thought I had just stabbed her horse with a sharp stick. He wouldn't let me touch any part of his right leg. I stayed about three feet away, still running my Reiki energy.

Then I did a chakra scan on him, maintaining my distance. Starting at his crown, I balanced each chakra as I went along. When I got to his sacral chakra, his energy spiked right off the charts and he jumped again. I finished the session from three feet away, knowing he found it too intense for me to be any closer. His guardian came back about three-quarters of an hour later and I described his stance to her. I asked her to come over and look at him. She didn't see it. He was no longer shuffling his weight or lifting his back leg and keeping it in the air like before. He was standing still, with all four feet properly aligned and evenly balanced.

Crystals

A great deal of jewelry contains crystals. Crystals are natural elements created within the Earth that all vibrate with their own unique energy frequencies. Animals are very sensitive to all energy vibrations, including those of crystals.

Crystals and crystal healing are not specifically Reiki or a requirement for you to practice Reiki. They can be a wonderful enhancement to Reiki and energy healing, so here are some considerations for using them.

You can find crystals at metaphysical shops or shows, gem stores, holistic clinics, and New Age bookstores, sometimes only for a few dollars. With crystals, larger is not always better or stronger. Find ones that are natural, not manufactured or dyed. Some say they should not be polished, that their natural state is better. I use both.

Horses prefer crystals or gems that have a very grounding (earth-based), low-frequency energy. In my day-to-day life, I wear moldavite or seraphinite on a necklace. They are very high vibration crystals, so I never wear them near a horse.

I rarely go to a stable with a collection of crystals in my pocket unless I have a reason to bring specific crystals. Whenever I am doing a session, I normally carry or wear some black tourmaline and/or some mookaite, for their very grounding energy vibration. Clear quartz is actually a high-frequency crystal, but it has such wonderful, gentle healing properties that it is appropriate to wear or carry anytime, for you or your clients. Shamans consider it the universal healing crystal.

You can carry crystals to provide their healing energy to a horse. You can hold them in your hand during the session, or they can be in direct contact with the horse. Again, be aware of how the horse reacts to the energy. The horse may find some crystals more appealing than others, and this could change from one session to another.

Crystals typically have the colours of the chakras. Any crystal whose colour matches a chakra will be helpful for the issues that are governed by that chakra. Horses are very connected to earth-based energies, so except when you are trying to treat something specific, stay with crystals that are in the red, orange, or yellow range.

Here are a some commonly available crystals that I would recommend:

Any "grounding" crystal such as black tourmaline (or any other colour of tourmaline), bronzite, granite, howlite, mookaite, red jasper (or any other colour of jasper), rutilated quartz, clear quartz, or septarian.

Here are a few I definitely would not recommend (these have a very high frequency):

aquamarine, beryl, cryolite, danburite, diopside, kunzite, kyanite, moldavite, peridot, rhodonite, selenite, or seraphinite.

Cleansing your crystals:

Crystals not only vibrate and emit their own energy frequencies, they also absorb energy from whatever, or whoever, is near them. If you choose to use them, you are best to cleanse them of unwanted energy regularly.

I flood mine with Reiki to cleanse them. Another way is to use high-frequency crystals. One of the best options is a piece of selenite. It has a high vibration and will dissipate any energy that vibrates at a lower frequency. You can get a small piece, hopefully reasonably flat. Then leave your crystal(s) on it or in contact with it overnight. You can likewise use a polished piece of selenite. In its natural state, it is like a collection of very thin glass-like strands layered along its length. Don't go running your hand across it—you'll end up with a bunch of painful, almost invisible slivers. Know that it is one of a few crystals that is water-soluble and will disintegrate if immersed in water.

Any high-frequency, high-vibration crystal tends to not need cleansing since it cannot pick up or absorb lower-vibration energy (it essentially just repels it).

I have always understood that black tourmaline does not need cleansing. It transmutes energy and dissipates it back into a neutral state. So, in the past I never typically cleansed mine, but I have since been told by someone that the one I was wearing needed to be cleansed. So now I do.

You can also cleanse crystals by leaving them in moonlight or sunlight. You can immerse them in dry salt, preferably sea salt. You can immerse them in salt water (again preferably sea salt). Only do that with ones that are not water soluble. The following crystals are all water soluble or can be damaged by water: angelite, calcite, fluorite, halite, hematite, labradorite, lepidolite, malachite, mica, obsidian, opal, pyrite, selenite, and turquoise.

Animal Communication

I am an Animal Communicator. Intuitive Animal Communication and Reiki easily complement each other, but you can do one without the other.

When you do energy healing, you get a deep soul connection to the animal. You may often pick up intuitive messages from them. Animals talk to us in subtle messages that may include words, images, or feelings. They can even be physical sensations that you will feel in your own body. You don't need to be able to communicate with animals in this way for the Reiki to work. Not everyone picks up on Intuitive Animal Communication, so don't let it worry you if you don't.

There are ways to tap into your dormant intuitive abilities or to enhance them. Everyone is intuitive, it's a natural ability. Unfortunately, in this fast-paced, commercialized world, many of us have forgotten how to connect to our intuitive selves. To tap back into this ability, pay attention to the subtle messages and thoughts that just pop into your head, seemingly out of nowhere. That's your intuition talking to you. Suspend your logical mind and believe what you experience.

I have made a lot of references to me talking to horses in this book. They do understand non-verbal, telepathic communication. They get it on an energy level. Animals are better at it than people are, as it is part of their natural way to communicate. Anyone can learn to do it. It is possible to talk to an animal just like you were having a conversation with a friend over coffee. There are many books and courses that teach it. Just like Reiki, Animal Communication can also be done from a distance.

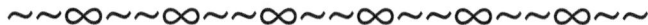

Summary

Crystals are often used by Reiki practitioners, but know they are not specifically part of Reiki. They can enhance your healing sessions, as can other healing modalities. You don't need them to be an effective Reiki practitioner. The same applies to Intuitive Animal Communication abilities.

Chapter 8: Safety for You and the Horse

While horses are very gentle creatures, and most would never intentionally injure you, you need to be aware of the potential for injury when working in close quarters with these large and powerful animals. You always have to consider the safety of both the horse and yourself. It is good practice to discuss the horse's normal behavioural patterns with her guardian. Ask them if there is anything you should know before the session.

One of the most important things to know about horses is that they have a blind spot directly in front of and behind them. When you approach them, it should be from a distance, from in front, and at an angle that is just off the front of their head. Never approach them from directly behind. They need to see you coming and know where you are.

Abused or traumatized horses can be a little more aggressive than the average horse. Also, horses naturally play with each other, and this play can include nipping. When they do this with each other it is just rough play that usually wouldn't seriously damage another horse. They may try to play with you in the same manner.

They do not always realize that this is enough to injure a person. You of course cannot allow this behaviour. All your normal horse handling behaviours have to kick into high gear. You have to demand their obedience. That may mean whacking them on the nose or sending them away, or you walking away, whatever it takes.

Always plan an escape route for yourself, but also provide the horse with one. Horses are flight animals. When they get the slightest hint of danger, their instinctual reaction is to flee. When I am outside and near a building or in a sun shelter, I always make sure I leave a clear exit route for them. If they dart for an exit, I don't want to be knocked over on their way out. It's not just the horse I am closest to, either. Even if that horse's nose is to the exit, there may be other horses behind that will want the same exit point. Anticipate the paths these horses will take if they need to rush to the exit, and be careful not to block it. You have to make it second nature to position yourself in the safest place.

You could be working on a horse with another one standing directly beside him on his other side, with their heads beside each other. If that one moves or spooks then yours could knock you over when the other one runs past its head. To avoid this, when another horse tries to crowd around yours, you are best to nudge yours over to create some separation between them.

When conducting a session, you should keep your feet pointed slightly away from the horse if you can. Don't face him directly. This makes it easier for you to step away if he unexpectedly moves his feet in your direction.

Do not walk or stay directly in front of him or under his head. When you are walking around a horse, make sure he always knows where you are. One of the best ways to do this is to keep one hand in direct contact with him as you move around his body.

When you pass behind him into the kick zone, walk as close to him as possible, directly against his butt. At that distance, a kick will have the least amount of force he can deliver. The kick zone is four or five feet in a half-circle arc around his hind leg. That is where the optimal force of a kick will be. Keeping close to his legs can limit the possibility of a forceful kick. Another strategy is to talk to him constantly as you walk around him.

When you disconnect physical contact from a horse, step directly away from him and at an angle where he can see you go. Avoid placing yourself directly between him and a fence that you could get pinned up against.

I do not recommend standing on a stool, bench, or any platform to reach any part of the horse. When you are standing on something, it is difficult to keep your balance and still move along the horse's chakra or body positions. A Reiki session can be like a wonderfully intimate dance, so you each need to be free to move wherever the energy takes you. For your safety, you may also need quick and unobstructed access to an exit route. Besides, you don't need any specific height to offer Reiki.

My Space, Your Space, Our Space

Boundaries. They keep you safe in every way: physically, emotionally, spiritually and energetically. With people, you need to establish healthy boundaries. Your physical boundaries keep you physically safe. Your emotional boundaries keep you emotionally healthy. Just setting boundaries isn't good enough, you also have to enforce them. It's not about being intrusive, abusive, or rude. It's just you establishing a line that is there to keep you healthy and happy. It's about self-care, self-love, and respecting yourself. You have every right to maintain healthy boundaries for yourself.

Having a physical boundary is an absolute necessity around a one-thousand-pound animal. Horses may need to be taught these boundaries, or taught to respect the ones you set with them. They need to know what contact you can allow, what you can't, and where. You can't let them push you around. Generally speaking, people say you should never allow a horse to move your feet. I have said that I will allow a horse to move me during a Reiki session. I think a better choice of words is that the horse "guides" me to where she needs me. I do not let horses physically push me.

As I have discussed, if a horse doesn't want contact, she will just walk away. People could learn a lesson from this. Horses tell me whether physical contact is acceptable to them and to what degree, or that they want the Reiki from a slight distance. We are in each others' physical space, but they also need to know what the limits are. I can't let them nudge me off balance just because they want to refuse contact and/or walk away.

The physical contact in a Reiki session is by mutual consent and mutual respect. There can be no dominance aspect to it, or else I don't continue in contact or even close proximity. I can allow a horse to lean into me for a firmer contact, but not move me when she does it. Sometimes I snuggle the horses but I always need to be aware of their acceptance and level of comfort.

After years of experience, the energy just tells me what is working, what isn't, and what is safe. I have a sense of what is happening between myself and the horse and the session seems to unfold as it needs to. However, I never lose sight of the potential for disaster. You must stay aware of the entire environment you are in. Never allow a horse to place you in danger or at the wrong end of a power or dominance dynamic. Either you get respect from the horse or you move to a distance.

Going Toe-to-Toe with One Thousand Pounds

Most horses who accept Reiki from you will stand still throughout the session. They can often shift their weight and shuffle their feet. If they are moving, then you need to keep one eye on their feet. Regardless of how much experience you have with horses, if you are around them enough, you will eventually get stepped on.

It's not a good idea to go toe-to-toe with a one-thousand-pound animal in your bare feet. I assume that you want your feet. A pair of boots with a firm toe is a requirement. No open-toed sandals. On that, most people agree. I say most people because I have seen stables allow open-toed shoes, sandals, and flip flops around their horses. That shocked me. Being stepped on can either just hurt or do serious damage, obviously.

The risk of being stepped on may be higher for us because we stand directly beside or in close proximity to a horse, sometimes for hours at a time. It's not like just leading the horse somewhere or tacking him up for a ride.

Now for the debate: do you need to wear steel-toe boots? You likely won't find a definitive answer; I haven't in all my research online, in books, and in conversations with experts. Some people say steel-toe cowboy boots are ideal. Some people say, "*Of course you should wear them.*" People at a tack shop have told me they are a good idea. Others say, "*Never!*" They say that, if a horse steps on your foot, the steel will collapse and cut into your foot or chop off your toes.

I know steel-toe construction boots are rated to withstand one thousand pounds being dropped directly on the toe. In their television episode "Steel Toe Amputation," the *MythBusters* team put the amputation myth to the test. They determined that it would take six thousand pounds to crush a steel-toe construction boot, and fourteen hundred pounds to squash a foot in a regular boot.[4] Other determining factors are whether the hoof lands directly on your toe, how long it actually stays there, and how much of the horse's weight is on that foot. If its hoof lands above the steel toe then the steel toe probably doesn't help anyway, as the hoof can still crush the rest of the bones in your foot. One other thing to know is that they can be heavier than other boots and are not as warm in winter.

I'll admit I still don't really know who to believe. I have worn steel-toe boots in the past but usually don't anymore.

Sunny Days

I am always happy when the pasture or paddock has some trees or a shaded enclosure and the horses are content to hang out there. You can lose track of time very easily when you are outside, dancing with horses. The hours fly by. Then you realize you just missed lunch or dinner, or both, and you have been in the sun the whole time.

The sun is always there, even when you can't see it. It's easy to forget that you can get a bad sunburn even on a very cloudy day. You can get one quicker from the sun's reflection off of pristine white snow in the winter because the sun reflects on you from above and below at the same time. A sunburn can develop in less

---

[4] *MythBusters*, season 4, episode 3, "Steel Toe Amputation," aired November 9, 2005, on Discovery Channel, https://www.discovery.com/shows/mythbusters/episodes/steel-toe-amputation.

than an hour on a day with a high UV index. My dermatologist tells me that nobody should ever leave the house without every inch of exposed skin covered in sunscreen, even in the winter.

Many adults who experience skin damage didn't get it as adults. The damage that appears in our later years was actually acquired as children or young adults. Most of us didn't understand the risk back then. I used to lay in the midday sun for hours when I was younger, and now I'm paying the price. That kind of damage can't be reversed, and it may come back to greet you later. So don't add to the damage that may already be there. Now I wear a hat whenever I am in the sun, and don't stay in direct sunlight any longer than I have to without sunscreen.

I have been told that sunglasses are not a horse's favourite thing to see someone wearing. They want to see your eyes. The same goes for hats that are pulled down well over your face. For your own safety this can't always be avoided. I wear transition lenses that change with the light. I also wear a hat, because my head has to be protected from the sun. I have found that once I am there and have made a loving connection, the horse starts to trust me and it works out just fine. They sense my energy and intention.

Can I Close My Eyes?

I am accustomed to closing my eyes when I am giving Reiki sessions to people. With my eyes closed I find I can more easily turn off the logical side of my brain and get into my intuitive alpha brainwave state.

Can you do this safely with a horse? The quick and dirty answer from horse experts is no, you probably shouldn't. You must ensure your safety at all times.

A horse will more easily follow your lead in their stall. Here, and in general, keeping your eyes open provides many benefits. It allows you to assess the horse's behaviour and body language, and to see the indicators that the Reiki is working. You will also see the horse move into you or away from you, as she directs the position of your hands. Her eyes will tell you what emotional state she is in, or if she is falling asleep. Ultimately, a horse who is happy with how the session is going will stand very still.

Subtle movements like muscle twitches can indicate that the horse is absorbing the energy, or it can be a muscle tone change in preparation for movement. I can feel her muscles twitch and predict when she is about to move. You can get to that place too, with practice. When I am in a stall, with a horse I know, and she is calm, I can close my eyes and just "feel" the session unfold. If the horse is moving her feet often, I will keep my eyes open and watch her feet.

Outside or at liberty, there are other considerations. If there are other horses within view, always be watching the leader of the herd. A horse will do whatever the leader tells her to. The horse's guardian may tell you who the herd leader is, or you can ask them. You can also watch the herd and their dynamics; it will become clear who the leader is. When other horses approach, watch the dynamics between them. The one you are with may welcome the approaching horse. Or not. It will depend on her position within the herd's hierarchy, or if she is in a sharing mood.

I am sure every horse guardian will tell you that whenever you are near a horse or a herd, always watch the horse or the leader. I do strongly suggest that you do that.

However . . .

I will admit I close my eyes during some sessions.

Only with horses I know well.

Only in their stalls when I am closer to the door than they are; alone with them in a paddock; or in a herd with the others well away from us.

Only once they are in a relaxed state and standing still.

Only with both of my hands in contact with them.

Because I stand in my Reiki bubble with them, an energy shift will tell me if something is about to happen. You have to be very aware of the energy to do this. I am getting pretty good at recognizing if a horse's muscle tension changes or energy level spikes. If you are totally in the moment, your touch will tell you which part of the horse's body is moving. You can feel every muscle movement and know where it happened.

As long as the horse is standing still, I can keep my eyes closed. If she is relaxed, she will usually have one leg cocked, with the front of her hoof on the ground, and that hip lower. When that hip raises slightly, she is about to swap legs. If the hip stays up, then she is possibly preparing to move. If you stay totally aware, you can touch the horse almost anywhere and know which part of her body is about to move. This is why I prefer to work on horses with bare hands and in physical contact whenever I can.

Even though I do occasionally close my eyes, I don't recommend it because it increases the risk of serious injury. Maybe I've just been lucky so far.

Your other option is to keep your eyes open and stare at a place on the floor or ground, with your eyes set to a soft focus where nothing is crisp and clear.

In a Horse's Stall

Horses are large and powerful animals. They are used to their stall being their personal space. I suspect they are not accustomed to anybody standing there sharing this space with them for an hour at a time. I don't imagine many guardians typically go into a stall just to stand there with them.

In a stall, it is easy for a horse to move and unintentionally squash you against a wall. You are best to always keep your access to the door open. Never have a horse between you and the door.

Occasionally I will move a horse around to get to his other side. Sometimes the horse seems to resist turning himself around and I will just stay on the same side. I'll admit that I have actually gone to his other side and had him between me and the door. I have only done this with horses that are relaxed and sedate during the session.

When doing a bladder sweep to complete the session, it is best if you can do it down both sides if possible. Sometimes a horse will shake off excess energy by flipping his head back and forth or shaking his body. His stall is likely big enough for him to move about if you tuck yourself into a corner when he needs to move. One more reason to have unrestricted access to the door.

Be aware that this can be the riskiest, most dangerous place to do a session. I have done this a lot, especially in my earlier (more naive?) years. I really liked working in a stall because it is a more controllable environment, as far as distractions go. I have never been injured; perhaps I've had luck on my side. A stall is an enclosed space. You can't run or push the horse away from you to get a lot of distance. You can be squashed against a wall if he spins unexpectedly. Regular workers have had that happen to them just being in there for a few minutes.

I don't normally go into a stall anymore. If the horse is on stall rest, I will just treat him from outside the door. For insurance reasons, many stables won't even allow you in.

Outside a Horse's Stall

You may be told by the guardian or stable owner, or just get the sense, that a horse is dangerous or aggressive. If you have any doubts about your safety, then do the session from outside the horse's stall. Reiki works just as well from a distance, and you will still see all the indications that the horse is accepting the healing.

One day I was treating a horse named Monty from outside his stall door. He was on stall rest and couldn't come out. The session worked just fine. I got one surprise though. When he was done, he walked to the back of his stall. I did the bladder sweep, on the side facing me. Once I completed the sweep on that side, Monty immediately flipped himself around 180 degrees to expose his other side for me. It doesn't get any clearer than that!

At Liberty

Your biggest concern here is to be aware of any activity around the horse that may cause her to startle and bolt. This includes weather activity.

Horses will be more anxious or skittish on very windy days. The wind masks their senses and makes them more cautious.

I have been told that they are more anxious and skittish in the winter too. The bright sunlight dancing on the snow creates highlights and shadows that appear to move. This effect is enhanced if there are clouds drifting by. Always remember that if a horse spooks or senses danger, her first instinct is to flee. Keep all exit paths open.

Some horses stay outside all year round. We can get frigid winters here in Canada. I bundle up in warm clothes if I am going to be in an open pasture, especially on very windy days. I do not pull a hood over my head though because that would create tunnel vision and block my view of what is around me. My peripheral vision allows me to keep track of all the horses in the pasture and their movements.

While Asleep

I am referring to the horse, not you. *Do not let a horse fall asleep!*

This is another reason to keep your eyes open and pay attention. It's OK if the horse has his eyes mostly closed or glazed over; Reiki can put him into a total Zen-like state. Don't let him fall asleep though! He could startle when he wakes.

This happened to me once when I first started treating horses. I had a horse with his eyes closed and his head dropping slowly to the ground. When it touched the ground, he woke up, startled and jerked, and his head bounced up, his eyes wide open. Then they immediately closed again and his head drifted slowly back down to the floor. Again, a startle response and a jerk when he woke up. He did this about four times.

The next time his head bounced off the floor and he lost his balance. He instantly hopped about a foot sideways to regain his balance and stay standing; I think he had all four feet in the air at once. Luckily, this hop was away from me instead of into me, otherwise I could have been picking myself up off the floor from under his feet, or have him crashing to the floor on top of me. *Don't let this happen to you. I never will again!*

If a horse is falling asleep on his feet, back off with the Reiki and ease him out of it with physical contact in an alternate position. Apply pressure with a gentle rub, a firm touch, or a nudge until you know he is awake and present. Then continue with the session. It's OK to put him into a Zen-like state, just don't put him completely to sleep.

I have confirmed this with a vet. If a horse gets startled in that split second just as he wakes up, he could jump sideways to get his balance, or he could actually fall over. The disorientation could be enough for him to spook and run. None of these scenarios would be good for your health, or his.

Horses do sometimes lie down during sessions. It can be amazing to see a horse feel safe enough to lie down and fall asleep in a paddock while you are giving it a session.

Here's where the safety issue comes in. If a horse lies down, you can't stay close. Move four or five feet away from his head; not behind him, at his back, or near his feet. Safety first, always. He will probably nap for about ten minutes. Then he will get up for a while, and then go back down for another nap. Horses may lie down after a session and have a little nap. The Reiki keeps working even after the session.

I don't have to tell you if a horse lies down in a stall, GET OUT.

When a horse starts to move his front foot forward, he is planning to get up. When the front foot comes forward that is your indication to move away, he's getting up. Horses can still go from lying down to bolting upright in an instant.

The figures that follow demonstrate horses lying down and sleeping in a paddock during a Reiki session.

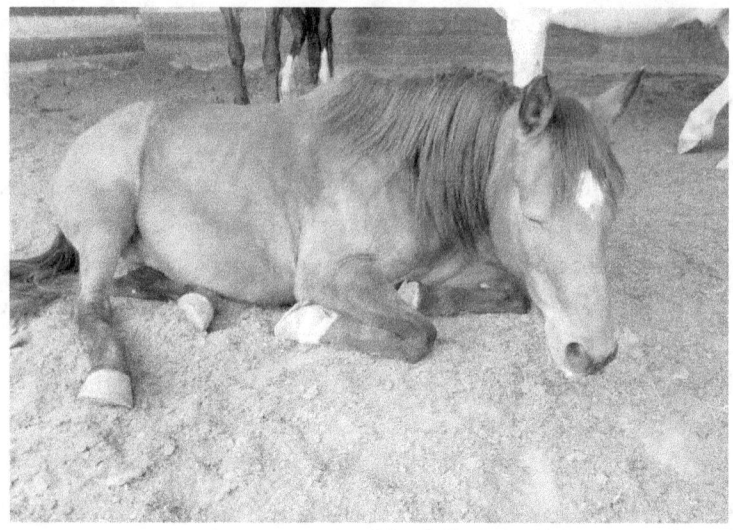

Figure 20: Buddy falling asleep

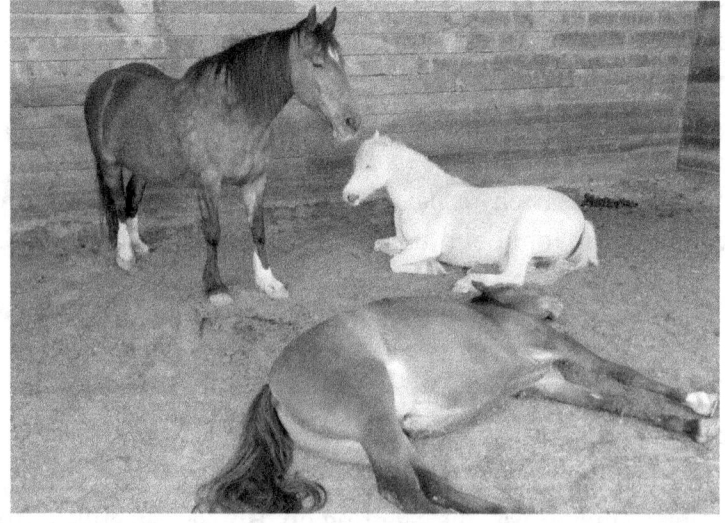

Figure 21: Milou decides to join Buddy for a nap

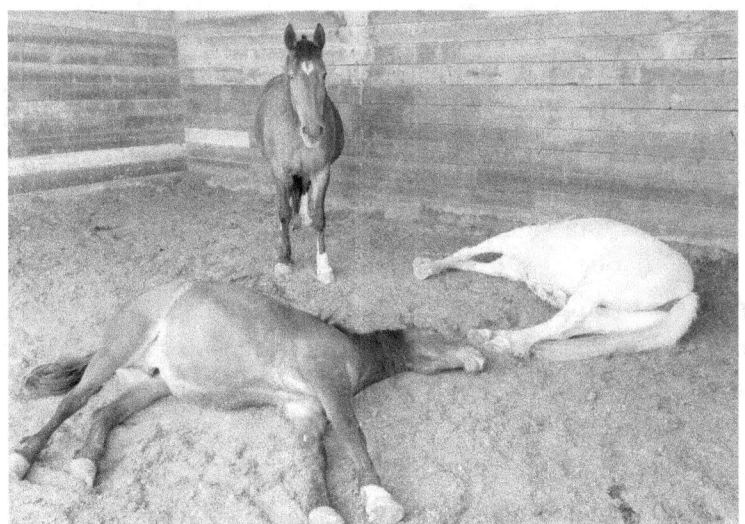

Figure 22: Buddy and Milou have a ten minute nap, Abby is relaxed but alert

When a horse falls asleep for you, like Buddy in this figure, stay just off the corner of his head and send the Reiki from four or five feet away. Even with your Reiki 1 you can send it that far. Buddy napped for about ten minutes, then got up for a few minutes, then went down again a couple more times. Milou joined him during one of his naps. Abby was very relaxed but remained up as their guard/protector. If one horse is down normally one will stay up and keep watch.

Bio-security

The industry is becoming increasingly more aware of the need for bio-security and procedures to prevent disease transmission. This includes any management practice that helps prevent the spread of infectious diseases from humans to animals or between animals.

Any movement of people or animals can spread pathogens between farms. Horses can contract contagious diseases that you would not want to have spread to your own horses or anyone else's horses. If you have your own farm with your own horses, and nobody ever visits from another farm, you don't need to be as worried. If all your riders or boarders only spend time at your farm and not with anyone else's horses, then you are less at risk. Taking your horses to other stables for shows or events, or hosting your own events, increases the risk. You will want to isolate everyone's horses from each other if you can. This includes things like their tools, water buckets, etc.

Bio-security is a topic unto itself. I won't try to document all the viruses, bacteria, pathogens, or diseases that can exist around a farm or animals. You do not need to know what they all are.

What you do need to know is this:

If you go from one farm to another, treating multiple horses, you need to know that you can transport contagions on anything that you wear or carry between farms.

My Advanced Equine First Aid instructor told me that the clothes she uses around her own horses only get worn there. When she goes to another stable, she uses other clothes and will wash them all before wearing them to a different stable. She will also disinfect all her equipment, all items in her first aid kit, and the supplies she took with her as soon, as she gets home.

A problem can occur just from walking through a paddock or stable where there are droppings. You get them on the bottom of your boots, then wear those boots to another stable. Do you know what you might have transported with you?

You will never get a perfect solution that eliminates all the risk. It is more about developing best practices that you can do daily and diligently to reduce the possibility of transporting contagions. It could be very easy to become fanatical about disinfecting everything every hour. I am not suggesting that, but you should at least be aware of the issue and create a workable routine for yourself.

Always wash your hands well before and after handling a horse. Wash clothing between different stable visits if possible. Try to find an outer layer you can wash regularly or at least wipe off well with some kind of disinfectant between stable visits on the same day. Not all winter coats are easily washable.

Decide whether to do your cleaning when you return from the stable or before going to a different stable. Do the same with any tools or equipment you travel with. It doesn't matter when you do this, just decide once then ALWAYS do it that way. No exceptions. Throw your clothes into the wash the moment you get home, no matter how late it is, or put them into a dirty clothing pile, and have another clean set available to wear.

One stable I frequent has a sign at the door of the barn saying they require people to clean the bottoms of their boots. The bare minimum you should always do is clean the bottoms of your boots and pant legs. Then spray the bottoms of your boots with a disinfectant, like Lysol. I leave a hoof pick and a large nylon cleaning brush in a plastic bin in my car to clean my footwear. I change out of my stable boots, and/or scrub the bottoms of them before I get into my car to leave. Nothing from my boots even gets into my car. If I am changing boots, the ones I was wearing get cleaned and go into the plastic bin in my trunk.

Find whatever routine works best for you and always follow it. If it is too complicated or takes too long, you will start forgetting steps, rushing through it, or skipping it altogether.

In the Age of COVID-19 and Beyond

The general guidelines above have been or should have been in place for some time now.

I'm hoping this section will eventually become obsolete. The novel coronavirus (COVID-19) pandemic turned our world upside down. Through the worst of it, the world's understanding of the virus changed constantly. Familiarize yourself with and follow whatever health and safety guidelines are in place at the stable you are visiting.

Some stables were scrubbing down all tack between uses and requiring masks in their barns. There has still been a debate going on as to the possibility of transferring the COVID-19 virus between people and animals or vice versa. I am not sure they have a definitive answer on that yet.

Some sort of virus seems to pop up in the world about once every ten years. I sincerely hope not, but I think it's safe to assume there will be another in my lifetime. Having your Reiki 2 is a significant advantage these days, since you can do sessions from a distance.

~~∞~~∞~~∞~~∞~~∞~~∞~~

Summary

Safety always has to be paramount, for you and for any animal you treat. Learn the characteristics of the animals you will be near. Understanding their behaviour makes you both safer. Always keep safety at the forefront of your mind. You also need to know how to keep your germs to yourself, to protect yourself and all your human and animal clients.

PART 4: An Understanding of Horses

Chapter 9: Introducing my Mentor

Carrington was my first equine client, my patient teacher, my mentor. He was also far less than physically healthy. Most sessions for a horse typically last for about an hour. I always let our sessions stretch into an hour and a half. Even after all our sessions together, he only once told me he had had enough for the day. Carrington and I learned and taught each other. He tolerated my fumbling around while I was learning how to do it, how to understand his messages, and how to interpret his body language. He became very adept at directing me to where he needed me. Or maybe more accurately, I learned to understand his directions.

When I was first learning, it once took me three times to clue in to what he was telling me. I was sure he had said yes to the session. I tried to start at his brachial chakra at his shoulder like I usually do now. He immediately swung his front end away from me and put his head into the corner of the stall. I waited to see what he was doing. He came back, so I tried again. Again his head went immediately into the corner of the stall. I stayed where I was and said to myself (and him), *"OK, I'm confused. I'm sure you said yes, so what are you trying to tell me?*" On the third try, the light bulb finally went on. He wasn't trying to get away from me, he was actually swinging his hip into me. I just turned sideways and laid my hands on his hip. Then he stood totally still for about twenty minutes and soaked up the Reiki. It took three tries to get through to me. This was all new to me and I was still learning. Eventually, I got it.

Carrington couldn't carry his weight evenly distributed on all four legs; one back leg couldn't carry his weight. Talk about a challenge. He would stay on one back leg until he couldn't anymore. Then that leg would release all his weight and it would shift to his other foot. He was constantly doing this dance while standing on a triangle of three legs. Sometimes he just raised his non-weight-bearing leg directly sideways for a stretch, then put it back down (an odd, unnatural movement for a horse). I got very adept at anticipating when his weight was about to shift and when a foot may come my way.

He was also the largest horse that I have ever worked on: about eighteen hands, so probably about eleven hundred pounds. I am five feet, eight inches tall and couldn't see over his back.

Other horses have stepped on me. It's inevitable when you stand right beside one for hours at a time. Whenever I approached Carrington, I asked him to please take care of me and to keep his feet on the floor. In all my time with him, every week or two for years, I did not get stepped on once. He did his best to keep his feet on the floor for me. I have seen many horses do this for me now, shuffle their foot across the floor rather than lift it to take a step.

On one occasion I was surprised to see Carrington stand totally still for an hour, since I think it hurt him to do that. He was always in some pain, but over time it lessened.

He always wanted physical contact. Over the few years that I worked with him, there were many occasions when he did a constant dance of movement. I normally treated him in his stall, where he spent most of his life. When I couldn't find a place to stand where I felt safe, he got his session from outside his stall. Near his end his guardian was afraid that if he were in the pasture and went down, he would never get back up again.

We developed a very special bond. Our relationship was a blessing. His guardian had provided me with unlimited access to my first horse client and let the two of us teach each other. I love win-win scenarios. I don't have horses of my own. This was my first equine client, and a case of Reiki for barter. He got unlimited Reiki sessions, and I got unlimited access to two horses to practice on, gain experience with, and be taught by. Carrington is physically gone now, but he will forever be in my heart.

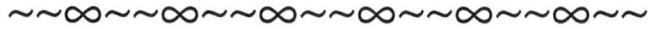

Summary

Meeting Carrington was one of the best things to happen to me on this journey.

Chapter 10: Understanding Horses

Horses have one predominant and finely tuned instinct for self-preservation, the result of millions of years of evolution: fight or flight.

Horses are prey animals. Their natural place in the world is to be another animal's dinner. No matter how well trained and controlled they are, if they feel scared or unsafe they will do whatever it takes to guarantee their survival. Their reaction will be one of fight, flight, or freeze. If they can't flee, they will fight.

To some people, their flight seems to happen in an instant. They will be right beside you and a split second later they are somewhere else. Their guardian may say *"I didn't see that coming."*

Prey animals live in the present moment. This is not how most people live their lives. Our minds are usually in the past replaying old incidents, or in the future worrying about what might happen next. Horses cannot be regretting yesterday or worrying about tomorrow. They stay alive by always being aware of what is happening right here, right now.

You are a predator. Any animal with eyes in the front of its head, who focuses both eyes at the same point, is a predator. You cannot approach a horse with the behaviour of a predator if you want it to trust you.

Horses have an innate ability to sense energy. They have historically existed in an environment where their survival depended on being hyper-aware of their surroundings. Even though the horses you will likely be working on don't live in that kind of environment anymore, their instincts are still there. They can feel your heartbeat from about three feet away. Horses often know better than you do how you are feeling. You cannot lie to horses: they sense you on an energy level, and energy doesn't lie.

When people are around other people, they often put up walls to shield themselves or hide their genuine feelings and intent from others, and their words and body language don't always match how they really feel. You can't do that with a horse. If your words or body language don't match your feelings, the horse will know. It will confuse the horse and cause her to be afraid or at least cautious around you. If this happens, she won't feel safe enough to accept Reiki from you. So, you have to be authentic when you are with them.

Since they sense all energy around them, anyone near them is also going to affect their mood. Any horse guardian can probably tell you that how they are feeling at the time gets reflected in their horse's behaviour. If they are anxious, then their horse is anxious. When you are performing a session, this can also include other people nearby, or the horse's guardian, if they are nervous about what you are doing.

Horses' Zone of Awareness

Horses have a "zone of awareness" that they use to protect themselves. It's their awareness of the energy patterns that they sense around them. People have one too, but many people don't know they have one, or aren't consciously aware of it. I am not talking about direct line of sight. When you are tapped into your zone of awareness, you are very aware of everything around you, of where everything and everyone is, and their direction and speed relative to your own. I hope you are in that state of awareness every time I share a road with you.

Our zone of awareness expands and contracts as needed. You can sit in a coffee shop working on your laptop and not even be aware of who is next to you or who comes and goes. This is perfectly fine if you are safe and the people around you aren't depending on you to keep them safe either. If you want to develop or enhance this awareness in yourself, practice always being aware of who and what is around you, regardless of what you are doing. Practice identifying where your zone of awareness is and how far out it extends.

A horse's zone of awareness similarly changes depending on circumstances. It may extend to the walls of the arena, forty feet past the walls, or even farther. The horse can't see what's there, but she senses it, or hears it. In a field, it may extend to the edges of the tree line. It will usually extend at least as far as the lead mare.

Energy penetrates everything, it is not dependent on sight lines. Your intuition and sense of the surrounding energy will help you determine where a horse's zone of awareness extends to. Notice the horse's energy field and find its outer edge. This can also show you how safe she feels. The zone of awareness of a terrified horse may collapse down to within a few feet from her body. You can help her feel safer by extending or expanding your own zone of awareness farther out than the edge of hers. That puts her inside your protective bubble and she will sense that. You play a protector role for her.

You can identify your zone of awareness by tapping into the awareness that your non-physical body uses to identify the energy near you. Your innate connection to the universe does this. Don't worry if this is an unfamiliar concept or if you can't figure out how to do it. It isn't necessary for your work with horses. Sometimes it happens unconsciously, and many people probably do it without even realizing they do. This is essentially the same thing as connecting to the energy of someone at a distance. You consciously connect to the energy of everything around you and become cognizant of how far that awareness extends.

Horses' Mental and Emotional States

Horses have four mental/emotional states: thinking, fight, flight and freeze. Below are some indicators to recognize the state a horse may be about to enter. I did say "about" to enter. A horse's first instinct is flight, and this is probably the most common response. A fight response usually ranks after that, when the horse's perception is that he has no way out. This is the **horse's** perception of his situation, not yours. Another instinct is to freeze.

A horse that is in "thought" mode is thinking and learning. This is the only state in which he can make logical decisions or obey a human's direction or commands. In the other states he is reacting instinctively; there isn't any conscious thought happening. Horses can't learn in these states. In "thought" mode they are much safer to be around and their behaviour can be more easily predicted, and, to some extent, controlled. They can bounce between any of these states swiftly (i.e., from freeze to flight).

Some indicators of a horse's state are:

In Thought:
- His eyes will be soft. If he is blinking, he is thinking.
- He will chew, a sign of being relaxed.
- He will have a relaxed tail.
- It takes about a ninety-second pause for a horse to register what he just learned and remember it.
- Looking at you means he is in the present and aware of you or your requests. His ears will be loose, soft, and relaxed, and his head lowered.

Fight or Flight:
- His head will be high, above his withers.
- His poll will be stiff.
- His posture will be stiff.
- Eyes wide open and staring is a fear response just like it is in people.
- Scanning the room with eyes wide open usually means the horse is under stress and looking for an escape route.
- Horses can be in flight mode while walking or with only slight movements; they don't have to be in a full run.
- They will fight when they perceive that they have no escape.

Freeze:
- If a horse perceives that he can't flee or fight, he will freeze.
- All prey animals do this because movement attracts the attention of predators. If they blend into the background and don't move, then they are harder for a predator to see.
- It may just look like the horse is asleep (or bored); he can't respond to any outside stimulus when he is frozen.
- His eyes won't blink or move around.

These are general indicators. You must take them in context with the emotional state of the horse, and the situation or environment he is in. All of it will influence his behaviour. Also, whenever you are near a horse, you become an integral part of his entire environment. Always assess the whole horse and the whole environment, not just one part.

When you are about to approach a horse, walk up slowly and stand still for a moment. Observe what the horse is doing and how he is feeling, and what is going on inside you, before you make any contact. Then approach the horse. Awareness of a horse's emotional state keeps us safer than just following any preset rules.

A horse's overall body and muscle tension is one of the best indicators of his emotional state. A calm horse has much less overall body tension; he has soft and relaxed eyes, soft nostrils, and a cocked (usually back) leg. He could turn his ears back softly just because his attention has gone there, without him actually being stressed. Ears moving around softly is just him taking in his surroundings.

A stressed horse has high overall body tension; eyes wide open without blinking; ears stiff with a lot of tension, or tight and alert (facing forward or back); tension around his face; and flaring nostrils. He will be standing erect with a wider stance and all four feet on the ground, with its lower lip pulled in tight against his jaw.

When a horse's body is this tense, it means his survival instincts are heightened and no logical thinking can happen. In other words, his is in fight or flight mode.

The term "fight or flight" describes a fear response that people often think of as singular isolated events they don't see coming. In fact, these reactions occur on a wide spectrum. When we understand the behaviours throughout the entire spectrum, we can better recognize what instigated the fight or flight reaction.

The spectrum leading up to fight begins as a brace posture before the horse escalates to aggression. The brace posture can just look like a stubborn horse that doesn't want to comply with your requests.

The spectrum leading up to flight goes from a head held high, to a head turned away, to bolting. The horse scans his surroundings to find an escape route; prepares for movement with stiff legs, wide eyes, and flaring nostrils; then he bolts.

The spectrum of freeze goes from "going inward" to immobility. It starts with eyes glazed over (where it seems like he's just not present), then breathing goes down. Then he becomes unresponsive, stiff and quiet.

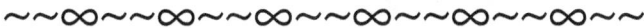

Summary

Understanding the behaviour, characteristics, and psychology of an animal will help you anticipate his behaviour. Life doesn't get much better than just hanging out with horses. Just make sure you do it safely.

Chapter 11: Herd Dynamics and Reiki

Can I Hang Out with Your Herd?

I frequent many stables where I just spend time with the herd, hanging out with them in a pasture, or standing beside them with my hands on them, giving them Reiki sessions. This is time I really treasure. It's precious. I find it enlightening to join them, as one of them, and watch their behaviour in a more natural environment. I am out there to "be" with them, not to be a human demanding or expecting anything from them.

It is a unique experience for both of us. I must be a genuine curiosity to them. I don't know how many guardians have ever spent hours at a time just "being" with their horses without doing, expecting, or demanding anything from them. Do they stand in a pasture just sharing their herd's company? How many stand completely still for an hour with their hands on their horse?

Try it sometime if you don't normally do this and you want to develop a much deeper relationship to horses. Join them in their world.

The first time I go through a gate to join a herd that does not know me well, I will see the leader's head come up and her eyes lock onto me. She is assessing me to determine if I am a threat to her herd. The rest of the herd will not approach me; they are waiting for her to decide. I then walk into the middle of the pasture, in a meandering direction, as another horse would do, and with no plan or intention. Walking in a direct line towards a particular horse, with my eyes locked on them, would be predatory behaviour or could be construed as my being there as a human to catch them.

I will not engage in any challenging behaviour. I stay about thirty feet away from them and stand still. The leader may just be confused: *"This guy walked out here, has no halter, and is just standing there. He hasn't even come near any of my herd. What is he doing here?"* It takes about a minute for her to make her decision, then she will ignore me. That's when many of the herd will come up curiously and nuzzle my hand or neck to say hello. It is their choice if they wish to approach me. Then they go about their grazing, ignore me, and accept my presence.

Few things are as relaxing and calming as hanging out with horses, especially if you are there with no agenda. If the horses approach me, I will touch them, but I do not make physical contact first.

Sometimes one of them will ask or even beg me for some Reiki. I will usually oblige, but this rarely happens when I don't go in with that intention or expectation. Since I don't offer it, they don't ask for it. I go out there to get a calm and meditative environment for myself.

My energy, intention, and behaviour will change in an instant if the circumstances demand it. I cannot allow their behaviour to compromise my safety. Since I don't challenge any of them, I normally don't have to worry about aggressive behaviour. I will quickly make demands of them if I need to, but it typically never happens when I approach a herd this way.

Don't be surprised if they don't initially know what to make of you. This will be a unique experience for them too. I think most people are too busy to do this. We normally walk in with an agenda, and the horses expect us to want something when they see us approach.

Normal horse handling requires a certain mindset. It has you approach a horse intending to catch him, put on a halter, lead him back to the barn, tack him up, and ride him. You walk into his stall, bring him out, put him in cross ties, and pick up the saddle. You don't ask his permission. When you are handling a horse, you just naturally exert your dominance.

Hanging out with horses is just not the same as normal horse handling behaviour. It is not the same as walking in with an agenda and demanding their compliance. That is a totally different energy projection and intention, and horses know the difference. You can't have an agenda, not even about how long you plan to be there. Just think of it as "me time." Most of us never get enough of that in our hectic lives.

If you do this, you have to give the horses time to adjust to new behaviour from you. This could really confuse or even worry them at first. They may have never seen you, or anyone else, approach them without an agenda. They could be saying to themselves, *"When are they going to tell me why they are really here and what they want?"* So, walk in with no plans, no demands, no expectations, no assumptions, and no time frame.

Maybe it's your own herd and you can't make time to do this regularly. You can start with short time frames. Just go join them and hang around for about twenty minutes. Do this often. They will learn that you are not always coming to make demands. It is also a great way to practice getting yourself into the perfect mindset for offering Reiki.

Try hanging out with them occasionally. You will love it. Join their world instead of making them join yours.

To Share or Not to Share, That Is the Question.

You might treat a horse while he is roaming free. If there are other horses around it can be an incredible experience just watching the other horses. When horses realize there is Reiki energy in the air, the herd dynamics can be amazing and hilarious.

The dynamic can take many forms depending on the personalities of the horses present. The others may try to get or "take" some Reiki for themselves. The one you are working on may choose to share it—or not!

If several other horses are roaming free, they will probably not run around near you while you are giving Reiki to one of them. They will either be twenty feet away or more, or within a few feet of you and standing still. They will soak up some Reiki energy for themselves; they know a good thing when they sense it. They could nuzzle up to the hind end of the one you are working on, to be in contact and get some.

The horse you are working on will either allow this or "chase" them away with a look or a nudge. You may see a kick directed at one of them. If he is in a sharing mood that day, he will let the others stay close or in contact.

It's not always the herd leader who demands their session first, like you might expect. The herd as a group will decide. They seem to know instinctively who needs it the most. Prepare to be entertained.

Here are a few examples I have experienced.

I was in the herd and had my Reiki turned on. I stood there for about ten minutes with my hands out, just offering it to any horse who wanted it. One gorgeous horse named Tina made a beeline straight towards me and stopped directly in front of me. I was amazed to see her spin herself around 180 degrees and back up about five feet right into my hands. As soon as she came into contact with me, she stopped. Then she stood there motionless for about twenty minutes, content to just soak up the Reiki energy I was providing. I was humbled. You will experience fantastic moments like this too. It happened so fast that I didn't have time to worry about an unknown horse backing up right into me, placing me in her kick zone. Energy warns you of things before they happen. I felt it was natural for her to be coming to me in that way.

On another occasion at this stable, I arrived to see horses who already knew me. I had told them I was coming. They were out of sight around the corner, in their shaded enclosure. I stepped through the gate and turned around to latch it. When I turned back, I was shocked to see all six horses standing right behind me. What an incredible welcome! Tina, who had previously "claimed" me as her own, started nuzzling my neck. The leader Charles started nuzzling the other side of my neck. The other four got the message that they were going to have to wait their turn, so they went back to their shaded enclosure. A few moments later Charles also left, and I realized he had left me alone with Tina. *"OK, I guess you get your session first—I've been told!"* This can happen often when there are other horses there too; the herd will decide.

In situations like this it is even more important for me to drop my expectations, desires, and any assumption that I know what is best, and to coax my ego into taking a back seat. I can't just approach one specific horse in a herd with the intent to give him a session, because he may not be the one who needs it the most. I can't assume that I know, or I will regularly get surprised. The herd knows what the herd needs because it behaves like a single entity. You can almost think of it like working on a person and having one of their chakra positions beg you *"Start here."* You get drawn to where you need to be in the herd, not necessarily to where you expect to be.

Later that day, after I had given sessions to all six of the horses, I prepared to leave. I turned off my Reiki, nuzzled each of them, said thank you, and told them I would be back another day. They stayed inside their shaded enclosure as I left. I was about sixty feet away, out of sight around the corner and heading to the gate. I stopped at a fence to offer some Reiki to the stable owner's goat, so I turned my Reiki flow back on, and was shocked to find all six horses standing right behind me. They had approached me so silently that I never even heard them coming! They know when energy is there, even from a distance.

On another occasion I was working with Dora. Shortly after I had started, I was surprised to find Tina's nose gently touching the middle of my back. Dora let Tina stay there for about twenty minutes, sharing the Reiki, then she kicked at her to chase her away, and was happy to get another half hour all to herself.

I have seen a herd of horses all share the Reiki, and I have seen them push each other out of the way and fight over it. Being wanted feels great, doesn't it?

It's not always the leader who "strong arms" the others into letting her go first, either. I went to see four horses in a paddock I had not been in before. I was told there were some herd dynamics at play there and to watch them carefully. The lead mare Belle would strong-arm (bully?) Riley. He was bottom of the pecking order and was having trouble fitting in. I knew this and hoped I could give him a session.

I made an assumption—remember what I told you about assumptions? Obviously Belle was going to chase Riley away and not let him have any Reiki, or at least not go first, right? Wrong. Belle and the others totally ignored Riley. I think they just pretend he isn't there, like he's invisible.

I stood in the middle of the paddock and turned on my Reiki. Then, as I usually do, I waited to see what response I would get from the herd. The other three ignored me and Riley came right up to me and said *"Me please."* So he got a session of almost an hour by himself, while the others ignored us.

Another assumption: he would want it on his root chakra, since he was having trouble fitting in and must not be feeling safe there. Nope! He wanted me to spend a lot of time on his crown and third eye. With my hand on his brachial chakra and crown he dropped his head to within a foot of the ground, his eyes were mostly closed, and his penis dropped. He stayed like that for about fifteen minutes.

I thought the lead mare Belle wouldn't want any. After Riley said thanks, I walked over to the other three horses. My Reiki was still running. Belle's eyes immediately got droopy, glazed over, and closed as she soaked up some Reiki. Zip's did too.

Then Riley came back for about twenty minutes more. Again his eyes were soft and half closed, and his head dropped almost to the ground. After this he placed his nose directly on my heart and kept it there. It was a wonderful "heartfelt" thank you.

Another time, I had a day when my brain was spinning. I was in the midst of planning house renovations. My brain was full of research, plans, checklists, shopping lists, and schedules. So many decisions to make. Among a bunch of other things also going on in my life, there was a family crisis happening. I was in the typical "monkey brain" mode. It all was keeping me from my normal sleep routine. Even my meditation sessions hadn't been very successful for a few weeks.

I normally go through life mostly calm and grounded, trusting that the universe will take care of me. I have my moments, like everyone does, but I usually bounce back to my centre relatively quickly. These few weeks were challenging. I debated going out to one of my regular stables just to spend time with the herd. How could I offer them any Reiki and have them accept it with my brain spinning its wheels like this?

Then I got the sense that I needed to go anyway, and that maybe we could help each other. So I went; just being with the herd has a calming effect on me. Sometimes I just go to spend time with them when I have a free afternoon. Maybe I wouldn't even offer them any Reiki. I was pleasantly surprised.

Many times, when I get to the pasture the horses notice me and then just go about their business. The moment that I stepped through the gate that day most of the herd ignored me, but I had three horses come to greet me: Lucy, Genevieve, and Grand Pacer. Lucy was new to the herd, and I hadn't met her yet. She walked right up to me and immediately turned my Reiki flow on! Did you know that can happen? Did you know that other people and animals can activate your Reiki and draw it from you, even if you didn't intend to offer it? This never surprises me. What did surprise me was that it was a horse I had never met before who did it the instant she got close to me.

I moved myself farther into the field, to a safer position away from the fence. The three of them stood there accepting the Reiki from me. I was standing with one hand out on each side of me, and had Lucy's and Genevieve noses in my palms. They stood there motionless. I was between their heads, a safe place to be. Any startle would have them each run past their side of me. This would be great if there were only two of them.

Now add Grand Pacer to the mix. A third horse adds a significant amount of instability and uncertainty; it changes the dynamic. What will the third one do? Where will he stand? How will he change the positions of the other two? Will he share or will he try to move one of them away?

Whenever a horse approaches the back end of another it is typically intending to move it. This can be different when there is Reiki in the air: they may just be coming to get some and the one I am with will not move away.

Horses will approach the one I am working on just to put their nose onto her rump to share in the Reiki. The one I am working on may or may not allow it. If she is in a full Zen-like state, she may just ignore the other one. If she is still in a very aware state, she may take the gesture as a signal to move away. So is the new horse coming to share, or coming to push the other one away to get it all for himself?

Grand Pacer stood near the side of Lucy and behaved himself. This was a case of "keep my eyes wide open." When they shift around, I can eventually have three facing me, with me in the middle of the triangle. That's the time for me to move to a safer position. Always be aware of your position relative to theirs. This worked fine for about twenty minutes. They would occasionally nuzzle each other, or put a nose under another one's head. That's a signal for me to move again, since this is an occasion where they may all end up in motion at once.

This is another example of why it can be harder to interpret body language and movements in a herd. I was standing at two of their heads, with one nose in each of my hands. Then I attempted to move in between their bodies and place one hand on each of their brachial chakras. It's something I have done many times while treating two horses at once. On this occasion they took my gesture as a request for them to move, and they both moved away in tandem. I went back to my original stance of one hand out on each side of me and they quickly came back.

On this day, the rest of the herd shared in the session on and off, three at a time. There were a few occasions where one of them would poke the other with their nose, and the horse would jump—prime behaviour to cause the third horse to startle and jump too. One would poke another or go nose-to-nose with him, which can also be typical challenging behaviour.

I had to cut off any potential for them to scatter with me so close. So I started talking to them, both verbally and internally, with a feeling and image attached to the message. The conversation went something like this: *"Play nice"* and *"Please make sure I stay on my feet."* The image in my mind was of them all standing still and me on my feet. Each time two of them would put their noses together I would point at them and say *"Play nice"* and *"You have to share if I am going to stay this close."*

This worked. They all cooperated, but I still had to stay very focused. I had to stay fully aware of where I was and of our constantly changing positions relative to each other. I always do this, but on this day they were making it impossible for me to allow my thoughts to wander. Whenever there are three in a dance like that, you have no choice but to stay focused. Each time another one would approach the pack, I had to re-evaluate where I was and where they all were. They shared well but kept themselves just frisky enough to demand my full attention. They came and went and jostled for positions. I was having so much fun.

For a couple of hours all my other issues and my "monkey brain" had vanished! My brain was empty of all conscious thought. Not one personal issue came to the forefront of my awareness for two full hours. It was almost like a great meditation session: I was totally in the present moment, completely aware of everything happening around me. They did that for me, gave me a wonderful two-hour break from all the issues going on in my life. This herd gave me exactly what I needed that day! Never underestimate the ability of a horse to keep you in the present moment.

Having a horse activate my Reiki happens to me often. When I walk into a pasture, I rarely turn my Reiki on right away. I greet the herd first and say hello to any horse that approaches. On another occasion I walked in and Lillian approached me; I had spent time with her before. I offered my hand for her to sniff, like I usually do. She immediately set my hands on fire! The instant she touched me, both of my hands felt like they were baking inside an oven. My Reiki was running at full intensity. The temperature outside was at the freezing point that day, but my hands were so hot I had to take my gloves off. You will quite likely have these experiences too, so don't let it surprise you when a horse turns your Reiki on before you do.

Just recently I went into a paddock with two horses. I had been there once before: one horse had been interested, the other had been very nonchalant about the whole thing. This time they fought over it. They both stayed within a few feet of me and in contact with each other the whole time. As soon as I placed my hands on one, the other pushed his nose between us and nudged us apart. So I put my hands on him. Well, didn't the other one force his way between us and push us apart. They kept vying for prime position. This went on for about a half hour.

They are a couple of real characters, very playful. When one wasn't separating us he would be on the other side with his head over the other's back staring at me, as if to say *"Hurry up, when do I get mine?"* Their antics were hilarious and I laughed my head off through this entire session. It's so much fun to watch horses when there is Reiki in the air.

Horses seem to very quickly figure out what is happening. They also seem to realize that being in contact with the one I am touching gets them some too, so I'm not always sure why they feel the need to fight over it. Being in my Reiki bubble (within five or six feet of me) gets them as much as being in contact with me. For the record, I don't mind having someone fight over me; everyone likes to feel wanted. I feel so relaxed, happy, and entertained when I do this. Besides, everyone needs a good laugh on occasion too.

Getting My Hands on Fire

The figures that follow show Fire and his bodyguards.

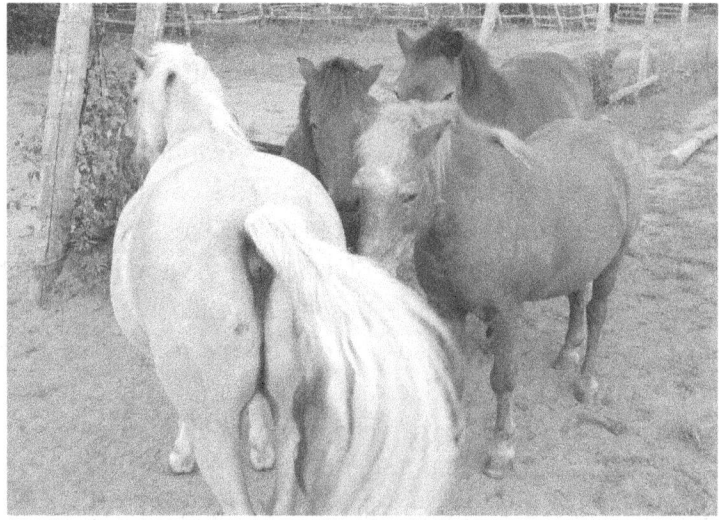

Figure 23: Bodyguards blocking access to Fire

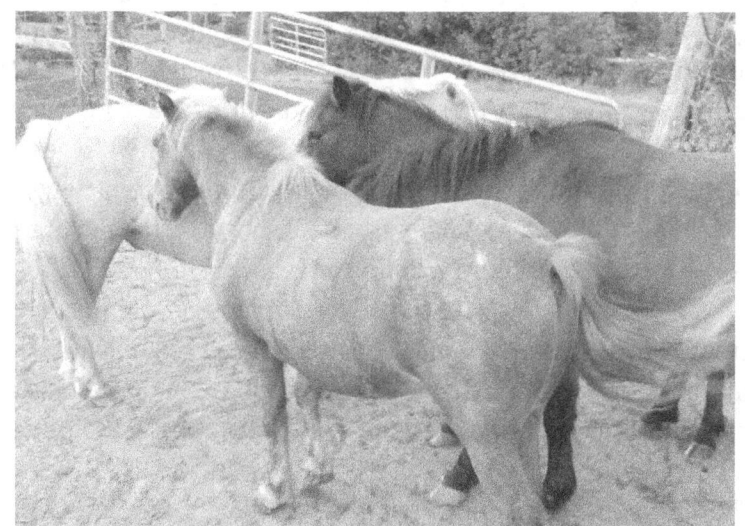

Figure 24: Bodyguards blocking access to Fire

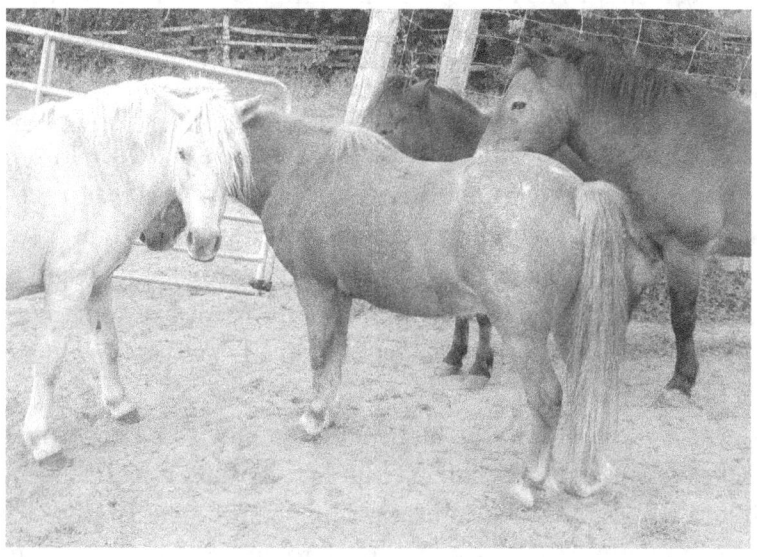

Figure 25: Bodyguards blocking access to Fire

Can you see Fire? He is the one back there, barricaded behind his three bodyguards, Morpheus, Checkers, and George. The first three figures show different protection configurations that they adopted. Like a security detail protecting a world leader, they were very adept at closing ranks to outwit my many attempts to penetrate their defences. Fire was soaking up the Reiki from the distance, and so were they, but there was no getting near him.

Getting my hands on Fire took a lot of patience. He was mistreated in a previous home. This horse gives a whole new meaning to the word "skittish." Even though we had many sessions together, I never got him to tell me about his previous home or what he went through.

The stable owner told me he had never caught Fire, and I never did either. Only the female stable hands could get close enough to touch him. They could walk into the pasture, put a halter on him, and bring him in. The herd protected him from all men. I was always amazed at the subtle dance they all did to keep me away from him.

I spent time in the pasture with this group regularly. I would run my Reiki energy from three or four feet away and see him accept some. This went on for months. Whenever I tried to get closer, the protection and avoidance techniques kicked in. A step towards him would have another horse appear between us, like it just dropped in from another dimension. Fire always kept another horse near enough for him to dart behind, always keeping one of them between us.

It was a game of cat-and-mouse. I took baby steps towards him over time, constantly reassuring him he was safe. Getting annoyed with him would have just reinforced his fear of men. It was a great exercise in patience. I was very careful to do this with no demands, constantly aware of his comfort zone. It took months before I convinced his bodyguards that I wasn't a threat to him. Eventually they stopped blocking me.

The following figure shows Fire's protection detail finally allowing me access to him.

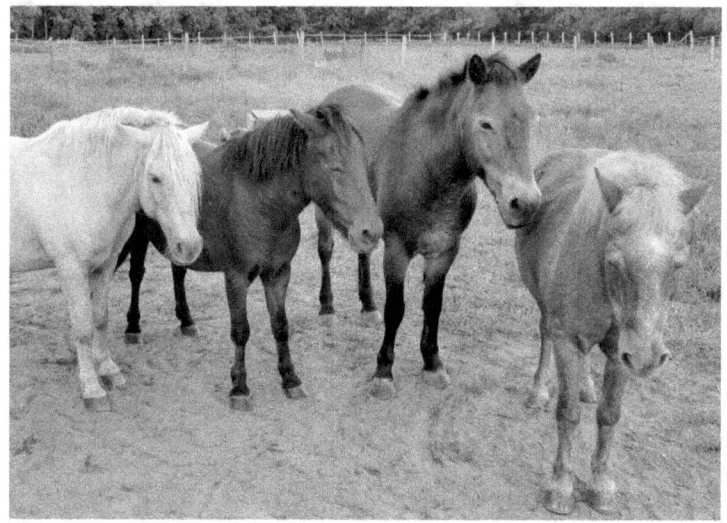

Figure 26: Bodyguards allowing me access to Fire

Then it was him and me. Over time, he let me get closer and closer. I could stand within a foot of him and let him take the Reiki from there. I couldn't try to touch him though, or he'd be gone like a shot.

The first time he touched my hand with his nose, I was elated. It was still all on his terms. I tried to move my hand up to touch his nose. Nope, not yet, he's gone again. After a very long time, he let me touch his head and shoulder. His guardian was amazed when he saw Fire actually approach me and touch me in the pasture. Fire's fear of men melted away enough to trust me to be the first man allowed to touch him. He was always much calmer after this, but he was never comfortable with any other contact from me, and I never found out why.

This is the most traumatized horse I have ever worked on. He is the only horse who has never let me eventually have full contact. Fire's story is a reminder that you may never get the result or answers you want, and you need to be OK with that. Just do the Reiki.

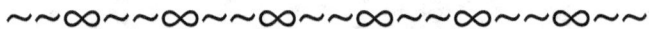

Summary

When horses get together, their antics can be hilarious. They all have their own personalities; and yet a herd will behave very much like a single entity, it knows what each of its members needs.

PART 5: Bonus Material for Equine Reiki

Chapter 12: Frequently Asked Questions

What Is a Typical Session Like?

There is no such thing as a "typical" Reiki session. Every session on a person or an animal is unique. What they need that day dictates how the session will unfold and how they will react to it.

I have described what some of my sessions have looked like, how I approach them, what often happens, and many of the similarities I find. Not that yours, or any future ones of mine, will play out this way. Whatever happens is meant to happen. People new to Reiki often ask, *"This happened to me, is that normal?"* Forget that question. If it happened then it is normal.

The horse will direct the session and decide how we interact with each other. Let the guardian know it could be as exciting as watching paint dry! Their horse and I could stand together totally motionless for an entire hour. Then she walks away and the session is over. Wow, that was thrilling! Then there is the other extreme.

The horse and I could be like a pair of sensual lovers floating effortlessly across a dance floor, oblivious to our surroundings. Both scenarios, and everything in between, are equality exciting for me while I am doing them. However, the first one can be a real bore for the horse's guardian to watch. You will need to reassure them that it actually worked.

Is This a Good Time for a Session?

Any time is usually a good time for a session, as long as it doesn't interfere with the horse's activity schedule. Just arrange the time with his guardian. A horse may have underlying physical reasons as to why it may not be appropriate on a particular day. A veterinarian should always treat any physical issue or injury first. In an emergency, you can start a Reiki treatment while you are waiting for the vet to arrive. We should assess extremely agitated horses, in terms of safety, before attempting any physical contact with them. See the section *"Safety for You and the Horse."*

Why Won't My Horse Accept My Reiki?

Getting some resistance from your own horse?
This can happen for many reasons. It may even be more challenging for you than treating other people's horses. Your horse will usually do anything for you, even if he might prefer not to. Offering Reiki is about the horse's choice to be in control of his own healing. Have you truly permitted him to say no to you? You rarely have the same relationship with other people's horses that you have with your own. It may not be the best time for him, he may not want it at all, he may not be feeling safe, it may be too noisy

and chaotic around him. He could also find the intensity of the energy too strong; he may want it only from a distance. Try to identify and correct the issue that is causing him to be unsure. Try to adjust the environment that he is in (i.e., location, activity level, noise, etc.).

If you are still getting a little resistance, or tentativeness, then go back to the basics.
- Check the surroundings to determine what is making him anxious
- Put yourself back into a calm mental state
- Breathe deep and slow (exhale with an audible sound)
- Drop your ego and any expectations or conditions
- Open your heart and make sure it is an *offer*
- Don't apply any pressure on him to accept it
- Hold an energy space for him and let him choose it

You have a couple of other options if he seems to want it but keeps backing away from you. Provide the treatment from a short distance. You will still see all the usual signs that confirm it is working. Your other option is to turn down the intensity of your Reiki energy. The section titled *"Wait, That's Just Way Too Intense!"* tells you how to do that.

I Am Really Short—How Can I Do This?

What if you are really short and can't reach the top of most horses to get to the chakras? You can still do this. Reiki Level 1 teaches you to go to each chakra position during a session. These are starting points, not requirements. Reiki 2 teaches you to place your hands wherever you sense they need to be and the Reiki will go where it needs to go. It also teaches that you can do a Reiki session from a distance, with no physical contact or even being close. So of course you can do this without positioning your hands directly on the chakras.

On a horse, most of the chakra points run right along the top of the spine. There are horses I can't reach either, but I don't have to. Reach as high up near the spine as you can while still keeping all your weight on both feet (for balance and agility). Placing your hands beside the chakra point will work just as well. You do not need to be directly on a chakra, or even in contact with the horse. Some horses can't handle the intensity of direct contact, and you will treat them from a foot or two away.

Are You in Pain?

I usually ask a horse if she is experiencing any pain or discomfort. Horses have a high threshold for pain and will tolerate a lot without ever showing you. What you may define as pain, they may only define as discomfort. It's all a matter of their perspective. So, I ask both questions and use a sliding scale to measure the horse's response. I visualize a ruler with numbers on it ranging from zero to ten. Then I ask the horse to show me on the scale where her pain or discomfort level is. This can be more accurate than asking her to describe it in words.

Just like people, every horse's pain tolerance level is different. I consider a three or above as significant enough to consider it an issue. I use this information to guide me to places on the horse that may require more Reiki. Severe pain could cause the horse to not want the Reiki there. I could try decreasing the intensity of the Reiki and closely watch her reaction to it. Significant pain is something I would tell her guardian about. My mentor Carrington initially gave me sevens and eights. See the section on *"Animal Communication"* for more details on how to have this type of conversation with a horse.

But I Need You Now, Can I Go First?

This is an example of why you shouldn't go to a stable with any preconceived notions or expectations of what is going to happen. On one occasion I went to a stable intending to treat two horses, Carrington and Howard. I planned what order I would do the sessions in. I believed I knew which horse would need it more; Carrington first, obviously. I passed Howard's stall, said hello, and told him I would be back in an hour to give him his session after I finished with Carrington.

I tried to walk away—it didn't work! An invisible force yanked me back towards him. I reassured him I would be back and tried to walk away again. Didn't work. Every time I took a few steps away, an invisible bungee cord tugged me back to his door. I couldn't ignore the overwhelming pull to stay there. That was his energy saying to me, *"But I need you now!"* It was a lesson for me to not ignore what the energy tells me. The energy connection between two beings can be that powerful. Howard got his session first, and I learned a valuable lesson.

What Should I Wear When Conducting a Session?

In general, you should wear comfortable, weather-appropriate clothing that you don't mind getting dirty. Also keep in mind that horses are curious creatures, and they like to play. Try to choose clothing that doesn't have any loose strings or decorative bits hanging down. Horses love dangling strings. You could find yourself getting choked if a horse grabs a string on a hoodie and tugs on it. A horse could also choke on the bob at the end of the string if he bites it off and swallows it.

Can I Wear Jewelry?

This is a personal preference. Many Reiki practitioners don't wear jewelry when they give sessions. I don't wear any jewelry hanging or in view that might get caught on anything or nipped at by a curious horse. If I wear a bracelet of crystals, it will be under a long shirt sleeve. I usually wear a black tourmaline necklace under a shirt. I don't show the horses any shiny object that they may want to investigate. Don't tempt them. The horse's safety always needs to be your primary concern.

Can I Carry an Umbrella if It's Raining?

It's best not to hold anything during a session. You need both hands free when doing Reiki, as they will often both be on the horse. You could need to hold a shank/lead rope and have the other hand free. You may need to open a gate and lead the horse through. You could have to push him away if he invades your personal space. I don't know of anyone who has or would take an umbrella near a horse. Certainly, opening one around a horse could spook him, just like any sudden, unexpected movement could.

Can There Be Music Playing During a Session?

Many of us play relaxing music for our human clients, and I've been told that horses like the same music as our human clients. Some barns will have a radio on, but I think it is for the worker's enjoyment. This might be an assumption, but I have always assumed that the horses would be happier without it. There is research that suggests radio causes stress for horses, and talk radio causes more stress than music does.

As prey animals, their senses are always analyzing their environment, and anything that blocks their sense of hearing could cause them stress. I have walked too quietly into a stable before without first announcing my presence or stepping loudly. This startled a horse when it caught my movement passing its stall before it heard me coming. It is standard practice at most stables to announce your presence by loudly saying "door" every time you enter. I normally always do, but on this occasion I didn't. Loud music playing can also mask your entrance.

I don't play music for the horse I am working with. I might try it some time, but I would keep it soft enough for only us to hear.

Music will not affect Reiki energy, but I sometimes find that music interferes with my focus. I can get caught up in the words of the song and start singing along. If the words of the song fill my head, how can I hear what the horse is saying to me?

If I am just doing the Reiki, this isn't usually an issue, but it can be if I am specifically trying to have a conversation with the horse and hear her answers. I will wear earplugs if I really want a conversation, especially when I can hear music from the other end of the stable.

At some noisy stables, I have even started playing some Reiki/meditation music on my iPod, with earbuds in my ears. It's not for the horse to hear, but as background music for me, just loud enough to muffle the words of the surrounding music. Music is also great for putting me into a wonderful meditative state. It's not safe to block all sound, of course, in case you need to hear something happening around you.

Can Two People Work on the Same Horse at Once?

Absolutely. This is common when you are doing a Reiki share with people. When I am channelling Reiki energy, I create a little Reiki bubble around me. When someone else enters the space, their energy blends with mine.

Horses are extremely sensitive to energy and can sense differences in energy patterns between people. If you know you are going to double-up you can do what is called "blending energy." Stand with your hands open and palms up. The other person faces you and hovers their hands, palm down, a few inches above yours. You will feel the energy pull between you. You will feel when the energy stops pulling and there is little difference between you. Now your energy frequencies are closer to being in sync. When you approach the horse, the energy between you two will be closer in feel and frequency.

Can You Draw Reiki Symbols on Horses and Other Animals?

You may often draw Reiki symbols directly in contact with your human clients. It is best not to do this with animals. They usually find it too intense and overwhelming. Instead, draw them in the air or on your own palms, then touch the animal. Always take your cues from the animal to determine what intensity of energy they are comfortable with.

What if Another Horse Unintentionally Absorbs Some Reiki?

Reiki expands past your own body and touches anybody that is near you. You create a bubble of energy around you. I often hear a horse in the next stall react to absorbing some of the Reiki I am channelling. I might hear licking and chewing, sighs, snorts, deep breathing, etc. As I describe in the chapter on herd dynamics, the surrounding horses can get some just by being close to you. This is how many house pets like it, with no physical contact.

The Reiki practitioners I have discussed this with agree that there is no ethical issue here. You intend to provide it only to the horse you are working on. Other horses may be close enough to pick up some energy from your energy bubble. You didn't offer it to them and did not intend it for them. They can also use their own intention to refuse to accept it; they won't absorb any of it if they choose not to. It's the same with your human clients. They have to agree to accept it; if they have no intention of allowing the Reiki to work then it won't.

How Do You Deal with Bugs and Insects at a Stable?

Some seasons there are lots of flies. So, why did your equine client just twitch? Muscle twitching is a very good, very clear, and very common sign that her body is absorbing the Reiki. When there are lots of flies, the twitching can just be her chasing away flies. So, some twitching is absorbing energy, and some twitching is chasing flies.

When there are a lot of flies and other insects buzzing about, be more careful of your foot placement because horses will stomp their feet to chase flies away too. Tail swishing can be to chase flies, instead of just to tell you what they want from you. You will also need to be much more careful if you are going to have your hands on their legs or feet. So, more flies require more awareness and focus on your part.

Recently I was in a paddock with two horses, Kasper and Nolan. They looked like they were dancing. Their feet were in constant motion. Every few seconds a foot would come up, kick their belly, side, or leg, and come back down. The energy I felt was akin to annoyance. I was unsure if it would be safe to get close to them.

I started the session from a distance and stayed there for a few minutes, then carefully approached as the session continued. Once Kasper accepted the Reiki he settled down. He got into a nice relaxed state and stopped stomping altogether, staying totally still for about twenty minutes. All the while the flies were still there. It's like he knew I didn't feel safe enough to get that close to him if he was stomping his feet every few seconds. As soon as he walked away for a break the dance of stomping around chasing flies started again.

Nolan stood close and watched. For some of the time he took some Reiki from a distance or by touching the other side of Kasper. He was never right next to me since we had Kasper between us, and his stomping dance continued the whole time.

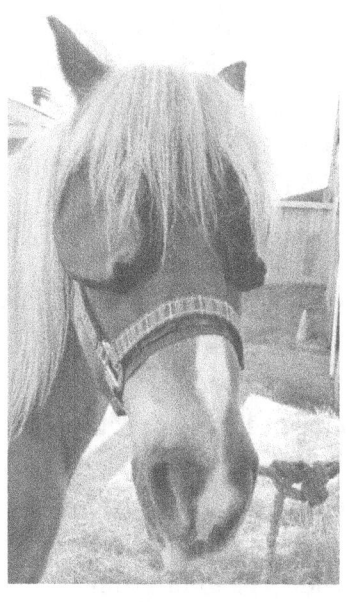

Figure 27: Monty wearing a fly mask

The other issue in fly season is fly masks. Some masks can make it almost impossible to see the horse's eyes. It depends on the type of mask, where you are standing, and the direction of the sunlight. If you are accustomed to always watching horses' eyes this can be more challenging for you. You need to watch for other clues as to how they are accepting the Reiki. I find this more challenging too.

This doesn't just happen at fly season either. I have worked on horses with eye issues or just sensitivity to light and who need to wear a fly mask all the time.

There will definitely be times when you will want to wear insect repellent, long pants, and long sleeves.

How Can Reiki Help Therapy horses?

Horses are natural therapists. Just being around them can have a calming and therapeutic effect. Many places in North America now offer programs in which horses act as therapy animals for people with various issues, like anxiety, depression, addictions, trauma, and PTSD. These programs involve creating a bond of trust between human and horse. They go by names such as Equine Assisted Learning (EAL), Equine Therapy, Equine Facilitated Wellness, and Equine Assisted Psychotherapy, to name a few. I myself am a certified Equine Assisted Learning Personal Development Coach.

When people go to an EAL session it's because they have issues to deal with. They may come to a session never having been near horses. They bring their anxiety into the session, which horses are excellent at recognizing and helping them with. Everything that a client feels gets sensed by the horse and mirrored back to them. This is why horses are great therapy animals and why this experiential learning environment is so effective at helping people identify their troublesome or self-defeating issues or behaviours.

Therapy horses are exposed to a lot of intense emotions that their human clients can find disturbing or down right terrifying. Although after a session horses are typically very good at dissipating any energy they don't want, I have been told that they sometimes hold on to about 10 percent of it for a while after a session ends. Some of what they hold onto can accumulate over time. Giving therapy animals a Reiki session is a wonderful gift for them. It can help them dissipate anything they picked up from a client and can help them re-balance their energy. Horses that do this kind of work deserve all the Tender Loving Care (TLC) they can get. What better way to help them decompress after a session?

Can Horses Be Reiki Practitioners?

Did you know you can attune a horse to Reiki? Then the horse can actually give himself a Reiki session, and can give Reiki sessions to people. Yes, they actually know how to do this. I understand there are a few places in the United States where horses have been attuned to Reiki. I haven't heard of anyone in Canada, besides myself, who has done it.

It was an incredible experience the first time I gave a horse his Reiki 1 attunement. I felt totally overwhelmed. It was for Carrington and I felt exactly like I was giving the attunement to a person. After I finished, I asked him to give me a Reiki session. WOW! I felt as though my own Reiki Teacher was giving me a session herself. Who knew it would be such an incredible experience, a horse giving me a Reiki session?

You absolutely must have their permission for this. Before the first time I ever did this, I asked Carrington for permission several times over a few visits. I wanted to be completely sure he wanted it. I also had to develop slight variations to the process. It's not quite the same as doing it for a person. You can't sit him down on a chair and lift his two front feet above his head.

There was no question in my mind that it worked. I know what it feels like to do an attunement for someone, and to receive a Reiki session myself. Having a horse give me a Reiki session was surreal. It felt bizarre to think this was a horse doing this for me. I had to remind myself that it is all just energy regardless of where, or who, it is coming from.

After he had his Reiki 1 for a while, I offered him his Reiki 2 attunement. His immediate response was *"Well it's about time! What took you so long? I've been waiting for you to offer."* I later learned that if you want to do this, just skip Reiki 1 and go right to a Reiki 2 attunement or do them both at once. Horses are so in tune with energy that Reiki 1 is almost beneath them (it's so close to their natural state).

What Do I Do When Nothing Works?

"I've tried everything, and nothing seems to work. I have followed all the guidelines and used every trick I've learned. She doesn't accept it, or it just doesn't seem to help." You may experience this.

It may be nothing you did or didn't do. Every living being has a life to live, a soul-purpose for their existence here. We can't change another being's life experience or destiny just because we want it to be different for them. We can't know what it is supposed to be. Try not to let those expectations creep in. Just because we can do this healing doesn't mean we are meant to fix everything or everyone. An animal's role may be to create that experience for her guardian or for herself. We can't change what that relationship or experience is meant to be. An animal may be here to teach her guardian how to love, and then how to deal with the pain of loss. She may be here to experience that kind of life for herself.

Reiki will always do what is in the best interests of the client, but it doesn't change their destiny. It will always have a positive effect on their life, but maybe it won't be something you can see. It's just like treating people. They may realize weeks after the session that something shifted in their life and you won't know it happened. You may see a physical or obvious issue with the animal and want or expect the Reiki to help with it. There may be an underlying issue that you can't see, that the Reiki will heal instead. You can't always see the result of a session.

This can be frustrating for us. It may be us deciding that we know what is best for the animal and then trying to control the outcome. This could be a lesson for us: to accept that we can't understand or alter someone's life path. Maybe the experience is to teach us humility. If we can't help the animal client fix what we have decided needs fixing, then maybe that is our lesson to learn from the session.

Why Do I Get Tired?

"Why do I get tired? It's Reiki energy I am channelling through me, not my personal energy." If you are always getting tired then follow the guidelines for preparing yourself for a session and for connecting to Reiki energy. Channelling Reiki energy itself will not make you tired, in fact it will energize you. Your Reiki 1 and 2 classes teach you how to connect to Reiki, and how to ground and centre yourself so you are just the channel for the energy. Your classes should teach you what sensations to expect so you can recognize when it is Reiki energy that is flowing through you.

If you do the necessary preparations and find you are still getting tired after a session, there are a number of possible causes. Doing any sort of energy healing work can be emotionally draining because you are connecting to a person's or animal's traumas and issues. You need to be well grounded and not pick up or hold onto that energy.

Prior to my retirement from my "9 to 5" job, I spent most of my life sitting behind a desk. It wasn't a job where I was on my feet all day. Now I find that just being on my feet for hours at a time can make me physically tired. You could be standing totally still for an hour. If you are reaching over a horse, you could be ever so slightly off balance (it happens, but try to avoid it). You could be crouching to work on their legs. Keeping your hands on top of a horse or above shoulder-height for almost an hour can be physically draining.

Doing a session requires a full hour of total focus and concentration (energetically, emotionally, psychologically, and physically). You need to be completely focused on your client, which requires effort. This may naturally cause you to become tired. Use this as a reminder to take care of yourself: you can't care for others if your own cup needs refilling.

Do I Need Business Insurance to Offer Reiki to Horses?

A few words about insurance and the love/hate relationship we have with it. We can resent all the money we pay for something we may never need or use. All that money spent and nothing to show for it. However, if we ever do need it, we will be grateful that it is there.

If you are going to treat horses there is a risk of them hurting themselves, other people, or you. They could react badly and damage something at the stable, like kick a door off. The stable owner could try to sue you for damages. You cannot always predict what will happen around a horse. If you want to charge for these services then seriously consider some type of business liability insurance. There are companies that provide this kind of insurance, for holistic and alternative healing modalities. The Reiki association in your country may have an arrangement with an insurance company for their members.

If you want to supplement your income doing this then what happens if you get injured? Will your basic government health insurance cover any significant injuries? Do you have basic medical coverage where you live? You may want to consider some additional health insurance to supplement what you have. At the very least, understand what coverage you do have.

Where Can I Find a Practitioner?

"Where do I find a Reiki practitioner for my horse or pet?" Reiki and all manner of holistic therapies are becoming more popular lately. It is not hard to find someone who says they do it. You can do an online search for Reiki, Equine Reiki, Animal Reiki, energy healing, holistic healing for animals, and so on. Check each practitioner's advertisement or website to find out what experience or training they have.

Many countries have a Reiki association. In Canada, the Canadian Reiki Association (CRA) maintains a list of practitioners on its website. The CRA requires a course certificate and numerous case studies to be completed successfully before the practitioner can make it onto their list. A person can't just say *"I do Reiki."* Not every Reiki practitioner in Canada belongs to the CRA, so this is not the only list of qualified practitioners in the country. Like any service, you need to do some research.

You may want the practitioner to treat your pet or horse in person so you can establish a face-to-face connection with them. You can also watch the Reiki being done and ask all the questions you want. It can be quite amazing to see how your animal reacts.

Reiki works just as well from a distance so you don't need to go to someone in your own city. It can be done from anywhere, by someone who has their Reiki 2 training. Your animal will still show you all the indicators that the Reiki is working when it is done from a distance, you just won't get to see the fascinating dance between practitioner and animal that I described earlier.

I find the simplest way to connect to a person or animal from a distance is to have a photograph. It is ideal if the photo has only them in it and their eyes are clearly visible. Whoever you hire for a distance session will very likely ask for a clear photo and the name, sex, and age of the animal. This helps identify the right animal to connect to.

Where Can I Find Potential Clients?

The best way to answer this question is to share my own journey. Not having grown up in the horse world, my journey to making connections in the equine world took many forms.

It all started with my first horse client, Carrington. That turned into just hanging out at the stable. The owner there was very open to me hanging around. He was very willing to educate me, explain things, and answer questions. We became friends. I helped with chores. That eventually led to me helping with the turnouts, bringing horses in, or walking them. I got to hang out and chat with farriers and vets, and I assisted vets with minor treatments. I helped with some lessons for the stable owner's beginner riders, teaching them how to lead, mount, dismount, give basic direction requests, etc. I availed myself of every opportunity to learn.

Being there regularly got me into many conversations with the stable owner, his workers (some of whom had horses themselves), and people who boarded horses or took riding lessons there.

I became friends with one of the boarders. She had just leased a horse named Honeymoon from the stable owner, who she eventually bought from him. When she was training Honeymoon, she invited me to watch and learn things like training techniques, groundwork, and lunging. She had a vet come and do a full pre-purchase evaluation. They were both willing to have me there. So I learned how a vet evaluates a horse, and I got to ask the vet lots of questions. She eventually moved Honeymoon to a different stable, which gave me a connection there.

As other horses were moved from this stable to elsewhere my connections branched out to those new stables too. I then took a couple Equine First Aid courses, followed by a beginner course on Equine Reiki and a few courses on Animal Communication, which gave me connections to even more stables.

All of this led me to taking riding lessons at a different stable, which allowed me to develop connections to the owner, the riders, and the riding coaches. The riding clinics there included instruction from farriers and vets.

I go to horse shows now. I exhibited at a horse show to introduce myself as a Reiki Master and Equine Reiki practitioner. I gave out some coupons for free Equine Reiki sessions. I also have flyers/brochures that I have left at many tack shops in my area.

Many of my friends and Reiki colleagues also have horses, so the connections just keep coming.

This is all to say that you will easily build connections in the horse world if you stay open-minded, friendly, willing to learn, and happy to lend a helping hand.

You also need an online presence: mine includes a website, Facebook page, and Instagram page. I carry business cards with me, and keep some in my car.

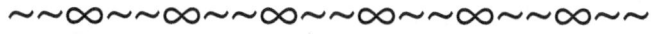

Summary

I hope I have anticipated and addressed most of the questions you may have.

Chapter 13: A Quick Checklist

I developed this checklist for myself when I first started giving Reiki to horses. I still occasionally look at it as a refresher. You can do some or all of these steps, or just use it as a guideline for when you're first starting out. You will eventually develop your own process that works for you.

I have broken the list down into very tiny steps, which are all defined in the previous chapters. It may seem very long and complicated, but once you have done this many times it just becomes automatic.

The Checklist:

- Arrange for the best date and time that will least disrupt the horse's schedule
- Connect to the horse and tell him you are coming (needs Reiki 2)
- Offer the Reiki to the horse before going to the stable
- Prepare your emotional and mental state on the way there
- Get out of the car and do a personal check-in
- Ground and centre yourself

- Clear your mind of thoughts and spend a few minutes in a quiet meditative state
- Quiet your "monkey brain"
- Leave behind all expectations and ego
- For horses you know, you may turn your Reiki on now
- Approach the stable
- Greet the stable owner or guardian and discuss the session
- Determine the best place for the session
- Set your intention for the session
- Clear the space you will use
- Ask for help from your guides
- Have your hands washed by this point
- Greet the horse
- Visualize the horse as being healthy
- Identify where your zone of awareness is and where the horse's is and wrap him in yours
- Offer the Reiki and wait for an answer
- Follow the tips for determining his answer
- Respect his answer
- Turn your Reiki on if you haven't already
- Stand close, but not in contact
- Wait for permission to touch him
- Start the session
- Gauge whether he wants physical contact
- Allow the horse to direct the session and determine its duration
- Let him know he is welcome to take as much or as little as he wants
- Follow the full process for doing the session (hand positions, doing the session, and when and how to end it)
- When the session is over, do a bladder sweep along his body, return his energies to him, and disperse all others into the Earth
- Pull your energies back to you and disperse all others into the Earth

- Disconnect your energy from his
- Thank him for accepting the healing from you
- Provide him with food and water
- Ground yourself
- Drink some water

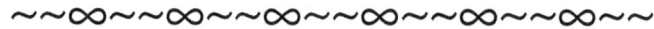

Summary

Here are the steps in a nutshell. Remember that these are just suggestions, not absolutes. Do whatever works. The most important points are being sincere in your intentions, making the Reiki an offer, and respecting the animal's decision.

PART 6: Treating Other Animals

Chapter 14: House Pets

Your House Pets

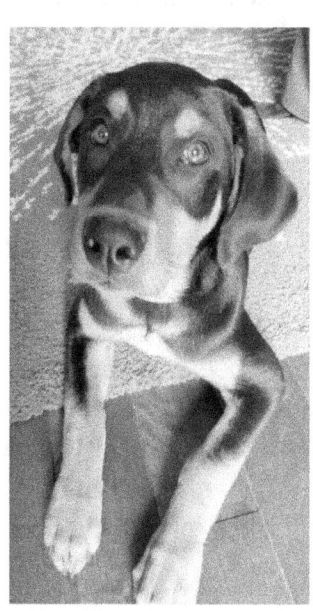

Figure 28: Freyja

Animals give us a sense of purpose. We take on a significant responsibility when we care for the life and health of another living being. In return they bring us so much happiness. They can relieve our stress. Their presence can help reduce loneliness or depression, and they are a constant source of companionship. They don't judge us for who we are. Dogs usually require us to walk them, which provides us with daily physical exercise.

Our pets live in our homes as well as in our hearts. They are exposed to everything that happens in the home. The environment we create for them (consciously or unconsciously) adds to their life experience. Any change in an animal's environment can cause anxiety or fear. A stressful house creates a stressful pet.

Pets can get ill or injured. They may have family members or other family pets come and go, temporarily or permanently. If a family pet leaves and never returns, the remaining pet may be afraid she will be abandoned too. If you leave for work and don't return for the day, your pets may feel separation anxiety. Your routine could change and they get used to you being home all the time, like during the COVID-19 pandemic. Then you go back to work and leave them alone all day again, and they don't know why. Reiki can relieve their stress and help them feel safe.

Animals may be rescues or have come from prior abusive households, or they may have been traumatized at some point. They may have trust issues with humans. You may bring one of these animals into your home and your heart. Reiki can help with their transition to their new home. It can let them know they are in a safe place and also help alleviate the pain of their prior traumatic experiences.

Reiki and House Pets

The content presented in this book applies to all living beings. What's the difference between horses and house pets like dogs and cats and hamsters and rabbits? All animals love Reiki. Even birds, reptiles, and fish like Reiki. They all have similar chakra positions, and the Reiki works the same on all of them. You approach them with the same intention. You still need to make it an offer, ask for their permission, and accept their decision.

The difference with horses is that they can inadvertently injure you, mostly because of their size, power, and being flight animals. They can't really sit in your lap either. Otherwise, most of the differences come down to each animal's unique personality.

Dogs and cats are extremely sensitive to the intensity of Reiki, just like horses are. Almost every horse I have worked on has eventually accepted some physical contact. Many dogs and cats seem to be happier to stay a few feet away from me or lying at (or on) my feet.

All animals require a safe and relaxed environment to accept a Reiki session. Clear the space of unwanted energies, just like you do with your treatment space for people. Create a loving and healing space for them to feel safe in. Their own home is where they will usually feel more relaxed because it is a familiar space. You or their guardian may want them in a room separate from any other house pets so you can minimize distractions. If this isn't really practical, you may be treating all the house pets at once. I recommend conducting the session at a time that least disrupts their schedule. Have their walk and meal finished.

With house pets, you are best to begin without attempting any physical contact. Just sit near the animal and start running your Reiki energy. You will be essentially creating a bubble of Reiki energy around both of you. Invite her into your bubble. Let her know she is welcome to come and take as much or as little as she wants. Then let her choose how close she wants to get to you. If the animal does come into contact, then you have her permission to touch her. She may sit in your lap or lie down on the other side of the room and go to sleep. You will see many of the same signs that she is absorbing the energy as you do with horses.

Much like horses do, house pets may come and smell your hand to sample the energy, move away, decide if they want it, then come back for it. As with horses, you can choose to enhance the session with crystals. All the same crystals and their uses apply to any animal. Follow the guidelines from the previous chapter.

For larger pets, you can touch all their chakra points as you do with horses, if they permit you to do so. If you have a large dog that is lying down, just do the side that you have access to. Don't try to roll him over; let him lie there and accept it from where he is. For a large pet the session may mimic one you do on a horse. He may move himself, or you, to get you where he wants you. I was once straddling a dog and working on her head. She was about eighteen inches high. She spun around and wedged her way right between my legs. There I was, with her between my legs and me facing her backside. I placed my hands on her hips and realized she had just put me exactly where she wanted me.

For smaller animals, if they allow physical contact, you can place your hands on their midsection for the entire session. Do what you do for every session: follow your intuition. If it tells you to move to another chakra point or to just stay exactly where you are, then do that. The animal will react much the same as a horse does; when she has had enough, she will just walk away.

Animals' reactions will vary. They do have personalities, and they have egos. The more a pet is around humans, the more she will develop an ego. Animals learn to manipulate their guardians to get what they want. They can be stubborn and resist even your best intentions. You will have to build some trust with them to get them to accept the Reiki.

When can you fondle an animal? Not always. Never try to get an animal to do something that she doesn't want to do. Don't try to force one to stay on your lap when she makes it clear she doesn't want to be there. It isn't respectful. It could also lead to aggressive behaviour. Do you like to be restrained or held captive?

Most dogs typically love to be handled, fondled, cuddled, have their bellies rubbed. Once you have their permission you can usually touch them anywhere on their body.

Cats, not so much. Newer research indicates that cats sometimes prefer people who aren't really "cat people."[5] This is because they may be more inclined to just let the cat do his own thing. Some "cat people" tend to want to fawn all over their cat, and try to keep him on their lap or snuggle him when he doesn't want to be there. Cats can be more aloof and standoffish. Or, put differently: they have strong boundaries and different levels of comfort. They decide when they want the attention and when they just want to be left alone.

Physical contact is different for cats. They have areas that they typically do not like touched at all, such as the base of their tail and their stomach. The research says that many cat lovers tend to touch these areas and can make the cat uncomfortable, while more experienced cat guardians don't do this. Cats love being touched at the base of their ears and under their chin. Their tails, legs, and along their backs are less preferred areas than their face.

These are generalities of course. Don't expect every animal to fit the same mould. Whether in a Reiki session or not, always be conscious of how an animal is reacting to your touch.

A Pet's Emotional/Psychological State

Animals are always somewhere on the spectrum between fight and flight. Their emotional state can change abruptly. A freeze reaction can just be them assessing the situation before they decide

---

[5] Joe Pinkstone, "Why cats love people who hate them," *The Telegraph*, August 6, 2022, https://www.telegraph.co.uk/news/2022/08/06/why-cats-love-people-who-hate/.

what action to take. A traumatic event in their past will still affect them in the present if the same situation arises again. They can have a physiological stress reaction to the same place, smell, object, or person. Fear can initiate a fight or flight response. While a horse's first reaction may be flight, dogs and cats are predators, so their first reaction is more likely to be fight.

Animals have all the same emotional responses to Reiki that humans have. They can also display playful reactions. They may get silly. Dogs and horses can do that when they are experiencing Reiki and deciding what to do with it. It could be a fear response or because they are confused about what is happening to them when they sense the energy.

Dogs and cats will typically give you clear signs that they are becoming scared, angry, irritated, or just plain uncomfortable.

A few warning signs you may see with dogs:
- Tightening of muscles or entire body tension
- Showing their teeth
- Growling
- Snapping
- Staring at you

A few warning signs you may see with cats:
- Extremely fast twitching
- Raised paws or extended claws
- Hissing
- Raised fur on their neck/back
- Dilated pupils

Always be aware of the emotional state of the pet and of her behaviour. You still have to remain safe. Remain aware of her body language and adjust the session accordingly. She could be telling you to get your hands off a particular part of her body. She could be telling you to keep your hands at a distance and not in contact with her. Animals are extremely sensitive to energy and may only want the Reiki from a distance. Constantly evaluate the messages you are getting from them; they will tell you what they need.

Ending a Session

You end a session the same way you do for a horse. The animal will tell you when she is done. She may get more animated or walk away. I have seen a dog voraciously gulp a full bowl of water in a matter of seconds after a session. She may fall asleep. Cats may begin grooming themselves. You may feel the energy connection dissipate. You may get the sense that there is nowhere else your hands need to go. With practice you just "know." Return all her energy to the animal at the end of the session and return your energy to yourself. Make sure you disconnect "energetically" from the animal at the end. Do the bladder sweep. Be sure to thank the animal for letting you do the session for her. Provide her with water to drink.

A Symbiotic Relationship

When we are in a relationship with an animal, we need each other. An animal and his guardian do not exist as separate entities; rather, their lives are intertwined. What happens to one always affects the other. It is a symbiotic relationship, also known as "mutualism." This may be more prevalent with house pets than with horses. We tend to spend more time with our pets; they even sleep in our beds. (OK, maybe some people do spend more time with their horses than they do with their family or pets.)

Animals mimic their guardian's emotional and physical state. They readily pick up their guardian's stress and have been known to sometimes adopt their physical ailments too. They are mirrors to our lives. When offering Reiki to a house pet, you can't remove the guardian from the equation. An animal's behavioural issues may be a reaction to what his guardian is going through, especially if the guardian is grieving. Sometimes a session for the guardian will significantly improve the animal's issues.

You can have the best result if you bring the guardian along for the journey. They need the same love, care, and compassion that you have for their pet. Judging the guardian for how they take care of their pet is not conducive to a successful experience for them or the animal. The guardian has to trust that you know what you are doing and that you have the animal's best interests at heart.

Reiki is wonderful for relieving stress in animals. However, stress is a symptom of a problem, not the problem itself. Helping with a symptom is not a permanent solution. If the initial cause is not removed, then the animal's stress will be back. An animal remaining in a household that is under major stress will just pick up the stress again.

These are relationships. How you treat the people or animals in your life determines how they will treat you, and vice versa. If you have an issue in any relationship, know you play a part in it too. Some animal behaviours are instinctual and cannot be changed. Some behaviours that are a problem for the guardian may be changed, but it may also require a change in the guardian's behaviour.

Sometimes animals will do something unwanted. They may be carrying major stress that they get from their guardians. They carry it until they just can't anymore. Then they have to do something to relieve or dissipate it. Their behaviour is them saying something is happening that they can't handle anymore. It could be uncharacteristic behaviour, like leaving puddles on the floor or chewing on slippers. The solution is to relieve the stress or the situation they are exposed to in the household; then the unwanted behaviour won't be necessary anymore.

If you do a Reiki session on the animal, you may pick up on some of the reasons for his behaviour. If not, the Reiki still worked. Effective Animal Communication can often get an answer from the animal about what causes him to exhibit these behaviours. Then the guardian can take steps to change the cause of the behaviour.

These may not always be comfortable conversations to have with an animal's guardian. You will need to be kind, caring, loving, and non-judgmental. You don't know their life experience. They may not know or want to know the part they play in their pet's behaviour. They may not be ready to hear it. If it's a behavioural issue they are asking you to help with, it's hard to suggest that a change from them may be the solution.

Energy healing is holistic. It is not compartmentalized, like modern Western medicine. It does not treat one system or one organ independently of everything else happening in the client's environment. We must always look at the complete picture of an animal's life and environment, and that includes the guardian.

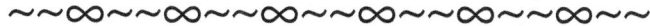

Summary

Everything you learned about doing this for horses applies to your house pets or any other animal, bird, or reptile.

Chapter 15: Transitioning/End of Life

This is the hardest part of any relationship with an animal. You love your pet with all your heart, knowing you will eventually have to say goodbye to him. The only pet that might outlive you is a parrot (they can live for eighty years). One of the most heart-wrenching things someone can do is to make an end-of-life decision for their horse or family pet. A common term for this transition is "crossing the rainbow bridge."

Reiki can help relieve the fear, anxiety, and stress experienced during this time, and can help with a smooth transition for the animal and his guardian. It can help the animal with any physical pain he may be experiencing, and reassure him that it is OK to leave. It can create a calm, loving, and accepting environment for both animal and human. It can also help the guardian with their feelings of guilt, especially if they made the decision for the animal. It can certainly help with their feelings of loss, sadness, and grief afterwards.

Animals are not afraid of death: it is a very natural and normal transition for them. Their guardian's experiences can be a very different story. We view death as an end, and we fear it. An animal will know when his time has come. He may stay longer because he knows his guardian is not ready to say goodbye. Sometimes an animal's reluctance to leave is because he is still taking care of his guardian's needs, to the bitter end. The animal is not afraid of death but may be feeling sad for the guardian he is leaving behind.

Animals do not go to the other side angry about the decision that was made for them. Sometimes they welcome it. They do not blame their guardian. Their guardian's depth of love for them is what prompted the decision and the animal knows that. They know the hardest decision of their guardian's life is made in their best interests.

You may be there to assist the animal and his guardian with this transition, using your Reiki. It is a Reiki session like no other, but still a Reiki session. You are there to provide what the animal needs, and that is a peaceful transition. You may be inclined to try to "fix" it. You can't. Your role is to assist the clients and accept it as a normal and inevitable process. You need to keep a wider, universal perspective on this. The guardian's grief and sadness belong to them. It can be really hard to stay disconnected from their grief so that you can create a calm, loving, and supportive environment to help them both through it.

When a family pet is near his end, we can often cuddle him during the transition. This is not always easy or possible with horses, so you may do the Reiki session hands-off.

What about the other animals in the home? Horses have their favourite companion. When a horse is near her end of life, all the other horses in the barn will know. When the horse is gone, the others will miss her and even grieve. After the horse's transition it could be helpful to give a Reiki session to her favourite companion. If it was the herd leader, the entire herd will go through an adjustment when a new leader is chosen. This can be very disruptive for the ones left behind. The same thing applies to family pets. There may be other pets in the house and they will go through a grieving process too.

Some experience with Reiki is a valuable asset if you find yourself in this position. Being well along on your own Reiki journey will help you stay balanced and grounded. It will also help you with the universal perspective of death as a natural process. I did not say any of it would be easy for you.

Regular visits to the vet are usually stressful for animals. Their guardian is probably right there with them for their checkups. The guardian is the animal's entire world, her family. When you take pets to the vet for the last time, they usually know what is coming. They know it will be hard for you, but they want you there. You are their rock, their life, their anchor. If you are not there, they will be looking around the room for you. They may be confused that you would leave them alone with strangers when they are scared, sick, and dying. You won't get any judgment from them for not being there, but they want you there. It will be their last opportunity to say goodbye to you. Just having their loved one there is a comfort for them during the transition. Reiki can ease their anxiety, and their guardian's too.

When the pet is yours . . . well . . . all bets are off. You are trying to support your horse or pet while you are in a difficult position yourself. You are overwhelmed by your own feelings of grief, sadness, and guilt. This is not the easiest time for you to be giving anyone a Reiki session, let alone yourself. If you can find the wherewithal to turn your Reiki on, it can help both of you. Meanwhile, you will be there trying and hoping you can fix it, or wishing you had done more. These are some of the most difficult times in life.

Reiki cannot eliminate your grief but it can help you get through it. Unfortunately, you have to experience the grief, and feel it, if you are to make it through to the other side somewhat emotionally intact. It is something that needs to be processed and worked through, not denied and avoided. Otherwise, it will continue to affect your life in many ways. Eventually you will remember all the good times with your pet and how much they added to your life.

Reiki can give you some emotional balance and peace, and smooth out the emotional roller-coaster ride that is coming. It can help you think more clearly and sleep better. Reiki can ground you and centre you, and it can help you remember that your life will continue. However, it is not an instant fix; there is no shortcut to grief's timetable.

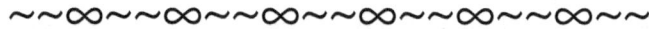

Summary

This is one of the saddest parts of doing this. It can be a real challenge to your ego too, wanting to help animals heal physically and knowing they won't. You become an observer of one of the worst days of someone's life. You can help the animal and guardian with the transition, but if it's the animal's time then you can't stop it.

Chapter 16: Reiki and Other Animals

Down on the Farm

If you live on a farm or own a stable, you may have other animals in your life like cows, pigs, goats, and chickens. They can all benefit from Reiki. I was once at a stable and was told that the owner's cow had stepped on a spike. The owner called the vet. While we were waiting, I offered the cow some Reiki. I put her totally to sleep for about an hour. Then the vet arrived and gave her some antibiotics, an anti-inflammatory, and a painkiller. This was a strange experience for me—talk about a stark contrast in treatment options. The vet woke her up from her relaxed Zen-like state to stab her with three needles.

Both treatment options were appropriate for the circumstances. You don't let a cow walk around in the muck with a hole in her foot. Reiki alone was not the best option for her medical health; it is a supplemental treatment, not a replacement for formal veterinary care.

Donkeys are wonderful to offer Reiki to. Their energy is so calm and earth-based. Their presence alone can put you into your own Zen-like state.

With farm animals, as with horses, you have to be aware of your own safety. I recommend that you learn or understand each specific animal's basic behaviour before you approach one. Learn how to be in close contact with them safely.

A head-butt from a cow can do some serious damage, or just really hurt. Cows are very heavy and much less agile than horses. You can't instantly push a cow off your foot like you can with a horse. A quick, forceful shove will have a horse jump sideways. I have done this to a horse before. I got him off my foot so fast that I'm not even sure he knew his foot had landed on mine. The poor guy was totally shocked! We were having a nice quiet and relaxed moment together, then I propelled him sideways. He wasn't sure what to do with me for a while after that. I had to reassure him that everything was OK, that I wouldn't hurt him, and that it was safe to resume accepting the Reiki from me.

At the Animal Shelter

You may decide to offer Reiki sessions to animals at your local animal shelter. What a wonderful gift that they could sorely need, but it can be more challenging for you emotionally.

These animals are often just discarded there and they may have issues related to abuse or trauma. They may need a lot of tender loving care. The animals may also have fear or distrust issues with humans. It can take a lot longer to earn their trust before they will accept any Reiki from you. So: patience, patience, patience.

If you touch on a shelter animal's trauma when you are treating her, it can be very disturbing to get a glimpse of what her life was like before she arrived at the shelter. Feeling sorry for these animals isn't going to help. There is one thing that may help you, and that is to understand that they got there by living their life purpose, their destiny. This is where they are meant to be. This is how they were meant to get there. As sad as it can be, their trauma or abuse landed them in that shelter for a reason. They could be there to find a new guardian so they can help each other heal.

You could treat some horses with the same issues. This is a good time to remember to accept that the session will unfold as it was meant to. Don't attempt to control it or even expect a specific result.

Wild Animals and Other Forest Creatures

If you live outside of a metropolitan area, you may have wildlife near you. Maybe you are lucky enough to have deer wander into your backyard. You can offer them Reiki too. Follow all the same steps you do for any animal: ask permission, end with a bladder sweep, etc. Again, a good occasion to have your Reiki 2, since you shouldn't be touching them. Get as close as they will allow and just activate your Reiki. You could be amazed that they will stand there and soak it all in, showing you all the usual indicators that they are accepting it. If you walk into the woods, sit quietly and activate your Reiki: you may find all manner of creatures come close and just hang around.

Lions and Tigers and Wolves, Oh My!

I have offered Reiki to predators at a couple of zoos. In general, it's hard to describe what energy feels like since it is a feeling and not something you can analyze with your logical mind. You feel it. You feel it with your heart. You can feel it resonate throughout your entire body; it makes every cell in your body dance. Energy in its truest natural form is pure love.

Even though their energy is still very loving, predators like large cats have a unique, very "primal" feeling to them. Their energy is so intense that I felt somewhat unnerved the first time I experienced it. They can be more "real," more "authentic" than domesticated pets, who learn to adapt to their guardian's wishes. This is nothing like your pet puppy. Domesticated dogs and cats are still predators by nature, but they live in our manufactured environments and have full contact with us. They are typically more docile than any big cat. Big cats and other large predators can never be pets. These are animals whose very nature is to be catching and killing their own food, not just walking into the kitchen to get it. Even in a zoo, their energy is very distinct from what you sense when you connect to a domesticated animal.

Try it if you get the opportunity and are so inclined. You will know from outside the fence that the animals are accepting it and that it is working. Having your Reiki 2 is what makes this possible, since you have to do it from a distance. You will get a feeling of calm, which can seem really bizarre coming from large predators. You will also get a feeling of gratitude from them after the session, just like you do from other animals. It's a "thank you" on an energy level, but it feels very odd and amazing to get that from wild jungle cats. Offering them Reiki requires the same process as offering it to any other animal: get their permission and follow the whole process from start to end.

Summary

All animals love Reiki; they can all benefit from it. There is little difference between animals when it comes to giving them Reiki sessions.

Afterword

A Few Parting Words

This is not complicated, really.

Offering Reiki to horses and other animals can seem complicated or intimidating, but I promise that if you give yourself the time and patience to develop your skills and intuition, you too can do this wonderful work.

I have included significant detail throughout this book. I covered some of the theory and background of Reiki, the process for treating horses, some considerations for what to do, how to do it, and many examples of lessons I have learned. Over my years of doing Reiki sessions on horses, I was keeping notes of what worked and what didn't work for me. I suggest you do the same.

I hope this book encourages you. Always remind yourself that you can do this. The Reiki will work, and it will even be your guide to help you while you do it. Don't overthink it, don't attempt to control it, just trust it. Understand that there is no right way, wrong way, or perfect way to do this.

All you need is to set the right environment for yourself and the animal. Start with the right intention and motivation (that you are there only for the benefit of the animal). Give the animal the choice of accepting it. Set your ego aside and follow the animal's lead. Stay tuned-in to what the horse is telling you emotionally and with her body movements. Remain present and aware of everything around you. Stay aware of foot movements. Be conscious of the entire herd's movements if you are not alone with the horse. Take care of your own physical safety. Stay emotionally connected, which can be difficult for you if you are picking up on emotional issues that the horse is releasing. Stay focused but also open to allowing the experience to unfold as the animal needs it to.

Forget about trying to predict or control the outcome. As they say, "just do it." Your horse will love you for it. You can't really do any harm with Reiki. This is not something that needs to stress you out, so have fun with it.

- Randy

List of Figures

Chapter 3, Energy and Chakras

Figure 1: Diagram of Equine chakra positions
Created by author. Copyright 2022.

Chapter 6, Doing the session

Figure 2: Zip in cross-ties.
Photo taken by author, at TrOtt, 2022. Used with permission.

Hand Positions:
Figure 3: Starting point at brachial chakra.
Photo taken by Kelly Poulin, 2022. Used with permission.

Figure 4: Starting point at brachial and heart chakras.
Photo taken by Vicki Bennett, 2022. Used with permission.

Figure 5: Crown and throat chakras.
Photo taken by Vicki Bennett, 2022. Used with permission.

Figure 6: Crown chakra.
Photo taken by Vicki Bennett, 2022. Used with permission.

Figure 7: Third eye chakra.
Photo taken by Vicki Bennett, 2022. Used with permission.

Figure 8: Encompassing heart to root chakras.
Photo taken by Vicki Bennett, 2022. Used with permission.

Figure 9: Heart chakra.
Photo taken by Vicki Bennett, 2022. Used with permission.

Figure 10: Solar plexus chakra.
Photo taken by Vicki Bennett, 2022. Used with permission.

Figure 11: Solar plexus chakra.
Photo of sacral chakra position.
Photo taken by Vicki Bennett, 2022. Used with permission.

Figure 12: Sacral chakra.
Photo taken by Vicki Bennett, 2022. Used with permission.

Figure 13: Sacral and root chakras.
Photo taken by Vicki Bennett, 2022. Used with permission.

Figure 14: Root chakra.
Photo taken by Vicki Bennett, 2022. Used with permission.

Figure 15: Working on a swollen knee.
Photo taken by Vicki Bennett, 2022. Used with permission.

Reactions:
Figure 16: Monty asleep.
Photo taken by author, at TrOtt, 2022. Used with permission.

Figure 17: Kasper asleep.
Photo taken by author, at TrOtt, 2022. Used with permission.

Figure 18: Chica yawning.
Photo taken by author, at TrOtt, 2022. Used with permission.

Figure 19: Chica with tongue hanging out.
Photo taken by author, at TrOtt, 2022. Used with permission.

Chapter 8, Safety for You and the Horse

While Asleep:
Figure 20: Buddy falling asleep.
Photo taken by author, at TrOtt, 2022. Used with permission.

Figure 21: Milou decides to join Buddy for a nap.
Photo taken by author, at TrOtt, 2022. Used with permission.

Figure 22:
Buddy and Milou have a ten minute nap, Abby is relaxed but alert.
Photo taken by author, at TrOtt, 2022. Used with permission.

Chapter 11, Herd Dynamics and Reiki

Getting my hands on Fire:
Figure 23: Bodyguards blocking access to Fire.
Photo taken by author.

Figure 24: Bodyguards blocking access to Fire.
Photo taken by author.

Figure 25: Bodyguards blocking access to Fire.
Photo taken by author.

Figure 26: Bodyguards allowing me access to Fire.
Photo taken by author.

Chapter 12, Frequently Asked Questions

How Do You Deal With Bugs and Insects:
Figure 27: Monty wearing a fly mask.
Photo taken by author, at TrOtt, 2022. Used with permission.

Chapter 14, House Pets

Your House Pets:
Figure 28: Freyja.
Photo taken by author, 2021. Used with permission.

Chapter Final, About the Author

Author photo:
Photo of author.
Photo taken by Cesar Correia, 2022.
Copyright belongs to Author.

About the Author

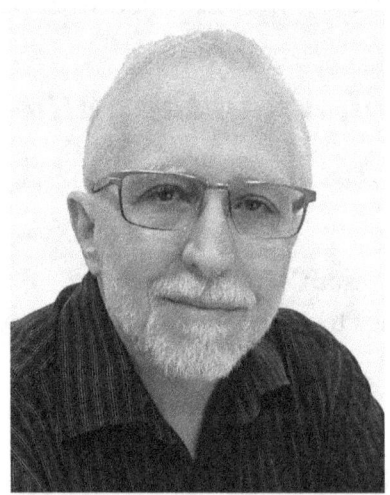

Randy Wilson currently lives in Ottawa, Canada. He grew up in southern Ontario with a menagerie of animals that included dogs, cats, hamsters, guinea pigs, mice, rabbits, ducks, budgies, pigeons, turtles, and even snakes. For thirty-five years he worked in the IT industry for a Federal Government Agency. After retiring, he was able to devote more time to his passions and quickly fell into Reiki and holistic healing.

Randy is a Reiki Master Teacher. After obtaining his Master Teacher Level, he began treating animals. He treats people too of course, although lately his focus has been on horses and house pets. After many years of doing Equine Reiki sessions, he realized that there was a need in his half of the province for someone to teach it, so he started teaching Equine Reiki classes.

Randy is a member of the Canadian Reiki Association and is certified as an Equine Assisted Learning (EAL) Personal Development coach. He is also an Animal Communicator. While doing energy healing on horses, he discovered he could hear what they were saying and have conversations with them.

Throughout this journey he has continued to enhance his knowledge and experience. He is on a path of self-discovery and enlightenment, studying topics on developing intuition and psychic abilities. His studies have included courses and books, different forms of energy healing, Shamanic training with the Foundation for Shamanic Studies, as well as numerous equine studies and riding lessons.

He can be reached at www.ottawareikimaster.com or on Facebook and Instagram as OttawaReikiMaster.

www.ingramcontent.com/pod-product-compliance
Lightning Source LLC
Chambersburg PA
CBHW071235080526
44587CB00013BA/1624